The Alzheimer's Diet

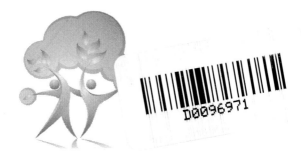

A Step-by-Step Nutritional Approach for Memory Loss Prevention and Treatment

JUMPSTART YOUR MIND JUMPSTART YOUR LIFE!

Richard S. Isaacson, M.D.
Associate Professor of Clinical Neurology
Vice-Chair of Education, Department of Neurology
University of Miami—Miller School of Medicine

Christopher N. Ochner, Ph.D.
New York Obesity Nutrition Research Center
St. Luke's Roosevelt Hospital Center
Columbia University College of Physicians & Surgeons

Publisher: AD Education Consultants, Inc.
Miami Beach, FL USA

The Alzheimer's Diet—A Step-by-Step Nutritional Approach for Memory Loss Prevention and Treatment
First Edition

ISBN 978-0-9831869-5-3
Library of Congress Catalog Number 2012949967

Follow us on Facebook! www.facebook.com/AlzheimersDisease
For more information, visit: www.AlzheimersDiet.com

Cover Design: Ciara Gaglio • www.cng-designs.com
Interior Design: Gary A. Rosenberg • www.thebookcouple.com

Contents

SECTION 3:   **What Should I Eat?**

SECTION 4:   **Special Considerations for Diet in the Treatment of Alzheimer's Disease**

Appendices

Acknowledgments

We are extremely proud of this work and excited at the prospect of being able to help educate some of the millions of individuals who have a connection to this enormously challenging disease. This book would not be possible without the help and collaboration of many individuals.

From Dr. Isaacson

A special thanks to my entire family, who have all played a significant role in my development as a person and as a physician. My dad was my biggest role model, and my brother my most significant career and life influence—I thank them both times a million for their love and eternal support. (Now if I could only get my brother to answer my text messages.) I would be remiss without thanking my mom (to whom I owe grandchildren, but now that this book is complete, I'll get right to it), my sister Suzee-Q, my sister and brother in-law Barbara and Mike, and my eight nieces and nephews.

To my mentors: Drs. Chris Papasian and Daryl Thompson (for teaching me in the early days of medical school and guiding my path since); Drs. Clifford Saper, Michael Ronthal, and Louis Caplan (for mentorship, training, and for holding me to the highest standard of neurologic care); Drs. Sacco, Pankau, Cohen, Zadikoff, Savitz, Benatar, Wright, Józefowicz and Safdieh; Ranee; Terry; J. LaRoe; the Helfner family; all my teachers/advisors at Commack High School (Jack McGrath, Ron Vale, and Dr. Doug and Susan Dreilinger) for setting the foundation of my education and future; my best friends Justin, Chris, Reza, Brett, Dave, Brandon, Mike, Jared, Harold, Tonnie, Janie, Steve, Peter, Dr. Andy Tarulli and Ricky's friend; Christine Greer; H. Ron Davidson; Dr. Sam Henderson; Nataly Rubinstein; Dr. Marc Agronin; Dr. Islon Woolf; Dr. Barry and Alyn Segal; Dr. Richard Mariani Jr; Carol and Gary Rosenberg for your expertise and ongoing support; Ciara Gaglio for cover design; The Regenerates (Ryan, Carlos, Marcelo, John, and Keryn), and last but not least, the N.Y. Yankees (for being the best sports franchise in the entire Universe!).

From Dr. Ochner

To my parents who continue to inspire me. Your unconditional love and support made me everything I am today and will be tomorrow. Thank you for not only being the most amazing parents but also great editors. To Dr. Robert Scott Ochner, the only family member to escape having to read this book several times. Miss you, Bobby. To my brother Ricky and sister Cheryl, you have both been siblings, parents, and best friends to me. Thank you not only for helping with this, but also for guiding me throughout my life.

To John Spychalski. You were one of the most influential components to my development, both personal and professional, and will always be a close friend. To Dr. Michael Lowe, for your mentorship, support, friendship, and proving that honesty and integrity are not preclusions to success. To Dr. Stephen Bono for being a continual mentor and friend. Your support and guidance are never taken for granted. To Dr. Eric Stice for being a role model and demonstrating just how much one person can do and achieve, while maintaining balance in life. To Dr. Xavier Pi-Sunyer for your continued support and guidance.

To the Irving Institute for Clinical and Translational Research (Drs. Ginsberg & Begg), the New York Obesity Nutrition Research Center, and the National Institutes of Health for supporting my research. To my outstanding graduate students from the Columbia University Institute of Human Nutrition, Dulce Barrios & Clement Lee. Thank you for your help, and I look forward to your contributions in medicine, as you will become outstanding physicians.

To my coauthor, colleague, and friend, Dr. Richard Isaacson. After all the sleepless nights, "work retreats," and "spirited discussions," I am extremely proud of what we have accomplished. The different styles we brought to this process have culminated in something very special, and the ability to create resources for helping others with my close friend is truly a unique privilege.

Finally, to my friends and girlfriends who have supported (see "put up with") me through this process. Thank you for understanding when I couldn't be there and for always being there when I needed you.

Authors' Note

"Tell me what you eat,
and I will tell you what you are."
—JEAN ANTHELME BRILLAT-SAVARIN, 1826

Following the success of Dr. Isaacson's most recent book, *Alzheimer's Treatment Alzheimer's Prevention: A Patient and Family Guide 2012*, it was apparent that patients, caregivers, family members, and even clinicians are actively searching for new approaches to dealing with the difficulties of Alzheimer's disease. In recent years, there has been an explosion in research on nutritional interventions for preventing and treating Alzheimer's disease. These interventions not only present new hope for people concerned about memory loss, but have rapidly expanding scientific evidence supporting their effectiveness. With Dr. Isaacson being a renowned expert in Alzheimer's disease and Dr. Ochner being a renowned expert in nutrition, the opportunity for collaboration between these two colleagues and friends quickly became obvious. The result is not only this book but also, more importantly, the nutritional program contained within it.

When it comes to Alzheimer's disease (AD) and memory loss in general, everyone can and should be using dietary strategies as part of a prevention and/or treatment plan. For decades, the medical community has recommended dietary management as part of the therapeutic plan for many other chronic diseases such as diabetes, high blood pressure, and high cholesterol. Today, those at risk for AD and those diagnosed with AD can adjust their eating habits to have a positive impact on their brains (and bodies) for years to come.

As a neurologist specializing in Alzheimer's disease (Dr. Isaacson) and a clinical scientist specializing in nutrition (Dr. Ochner), our daily efforts are focused on three areas: patient care, research, and education. We teach other physicians and PhDs, as well as medical and graduate students, at two large and well-respected academic medical centers in the United States. We work closely with and help educate doctors, scientists, psychologists, nurses, nurse practitioners, trainees, and other members of the healthcare team.

Regardless of the audiences to which we have spoken, we have found a significant gap between potential interventions for Alzheimer's disease and what is actually recommended to patients. This gap in treatment, as well as the personal experiences of our family members, patients, and close friends, prompted us to write this book.

In this book, we present all we have learned through our training and clinical practice. We also discuss our real-life experiences in suggesting dietary modification to patients, caregivers, family members, clients, and television and radio audiences. We have studied the scientific literature, published medical journal articles, and presented our research at conferences throughout the world. This book is a summation of the science behind AD nutrition and the experience we have gained in applying this knowledge over the last fifteen years.

The Alzheimer's Diet includes excerpts from the scientific literature that will benefit treating physicians and other medical providers. However, we also translate this information to be understandable for people with Alzheimer's disease as well as their caretakers and family members. While we do use technical terms, such as "beta-amyloid peptides" and "nutrigenomics," we do our best to avoid overusing them. You will not need an advanced course or medical degree to understand these terms, but we do include them for medical professionals who will also be reading. It is our goal to present this vital information in a way that anyone can apply specific concepts toward better brain health.

There are several ways to look at our overall philosophy of treating and preventing Alzheimer's disease through diet. As a result of personal experiences and a family history of Alzheimer's disease, Dr. Isaacson treats his patients exactly the same as he would treat his own family members. In his clinical practice, as in this book, considerations are made by weighing the risk-benefit ratio of interventions. If the risk is low and potential for benefit is moderate or high, we suggest it.

As you continue to expand your knowledge and understanding of Alzheimer's nutrition, remember the saying, "Rome wasn't built in a day." At first, choose a few aspects on which to focus. Start slowly and realize that efforts now will be rewarded later. There is no better investment than in the health of oneself or in the ones we care about!

—Christopher N. Ochner, Ph.D.
& Richard S. Isaacson, M.D.

Author Disclosure: Dr. Isaacson has served as a paid scientific advisor/consultant for companies that sell the FDA-approved cholinesterase inhibitor medications and the FDA-regulated medical food. Drs. Isaacson and Ochner have served as scientific advisors for therapyformemory.org.

Introduction

PART 1—THE ALZHEIMER'S DIET OVERVIEW

"Although there is a great deal of controversy among scientists about the effects of ingested food on the brain, no one denies that you can change your cognition and mood by what you eat."

—ARTHUR HENRY WINTER (1844–1937)

At any moment, anyone can start to make changes in his or her diet that benefit health, boost memory, and improve the ability to fight Alzheimer's disease (AD). This book is based on the latest scientific research and will teach you what you need to know about diet and nutrition in order to achieve these benefits.

The Problem: Over time, certain foods and beverages can interfere with memory function.

The Solution: Education and guidance! *The Alzheimer's Diet* is a detailed how-to guide on making brain-healthy food choices without sacrificing favorite foods.

1

The Alzheimer's Diet details dietary and nutrition strategies that we have shared with our patients, as well as our own family members, to help them protect memory function and optimize brain health. In addition to providing practical examples of how these people have succeeded, we review the most common obstacles encountered and outline specific strategies to overcome them. In Section 1, we begin by providing fundamental background information on the relationship between diet and brain function. In Section 2, we address how this information can be put into action in order to improve memory and overall brain health. In Section 3, we guide you through the detailed step-by-step 9-Week Diet Plan approach and provided practical guides for grocery shopping and restaurant eating.

As a part of the 9-Week Diet Plan (see Chapter 18), we recommend that you track and record relevant information in order to assist with adopting a brain-healthy diet. We provide space to record this information in the back of the book (see Appendix F) but also offer an online tool to record and store this information electronically. For access to the innovative online **Alzheimer's Disease—Nutrition Tracking System (AD-NTS™)**, go to www.AlzheimersDiet.com.

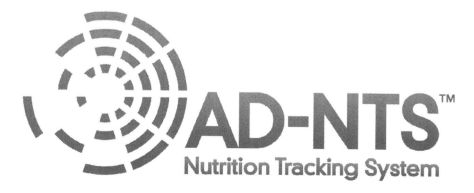

The AD-NTS™ system enables the user to track essential brain-healthy diet information, such as food and macronutrient intake (carbohydrates, fat, and protein), brain-healthy foods and recipes, body markers (weight and blood pressure), laboratory results, medications, medical foods, vitamins, supplements, and lifestyle activities (physical and mental exercise).

AD-NTS™ Components:

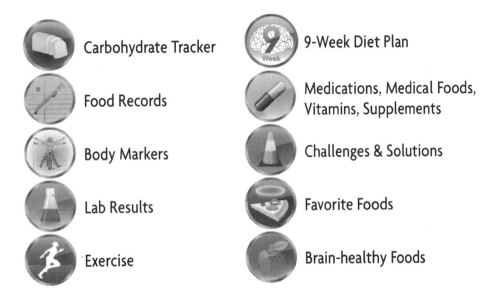

Carbohydrate Tracker

9-Week Diet Plan

Food Records

Medications, Medical Foods, Vitamins, Supplements

Body Markers

Challenges & Solutions

Lab Results

Favorite Foods

Exercise

Brain-healthy Foods

The AD-NTS includes specific week-by-week tracking metrics such as recording of favorite brain-unhealthy snacks and meals to be adapted or substituted, as well as Challenges and Potential Solutions to brain-healthy eating. Customized reports can be printed, which help track progress as well as make it easy to communicate information at doctor's visits and nutrition consultations.

In this book, we focus on maximizing the potential for success. We believe that a step-wise approach toward dietary change works best. Everyone should start off successfully with the 9-Week Diet Plan since absolutely no changes should be made to foods eaten in the first week. Instead, the first week focuses on learning about the effects of diet and nutrition on AD and preparing for changes to come. This is followed by learning how to read and analyze nutrition labels. The next essential step is to apply that knowledge when purchasing food and eating out.

In Section 4, we address special considerations related to the treatment of Alzheimer's disease. For example, we will discuss why certain strategies may work better for some individuals more than others.

Throughout the book, we provide detailed explanations of all key areas of brain-healthy diet and nutrition (e.g., food ingredients, nutrients, understanding nutrition labels, antioxidants, meal replacements, 12–14 hour fasting, coffee and other caffeinated beverages, vitamins, supplements, medical foods, effect of genetics on food response, and multicultural considerations). Readers will become knowledgeable about how particular food choices may, over time, either delay the onset of AD or improve memory function in patients already diagnosed with AD. Readers will also learn which foods to avoid; those that can actually *increase* the likelihood of developing AD, as well as cause AD symptoms to worsen. More importantly, readers will learn how to apply this knowledge and immediately begin making dietary changes that can have a large impact on memory function and overall quality of life.

ESSENTIAL CONCEPTS OF THE ALZHEIMER'S DIET

One of the core principles of the Alzheimer's Diet relates to specific nutrients, called macronutrients. Fat, protein, and carbohydrate are the main macronutrients, which we will discuss in Chapters 9, 10, and 11. In these chapters, we also provide specific examples of healthy and unhealthy macronutrient selections.

DEFINITION: Macronutrients

Nutrients required in relatively large amounts for the proper growth, development, and functioning of an organism. The major macronutrients include fat, protein, carbohydrate, and water.

The following are general recommendations for macronutrients in Alzheimer's nutrition:

1. Decrease carbohydrates in general but, more specifically, minimize specific types and amounts that significantly and rapidly raise blood sugar. Carbohydrates include foods like bread, cereal, and sugar. Different types of carbs are more harmful to the brain than others.

2. Decrease saturated fats, and select the right types of healthy and brain-protective fats (e.g., specific Omega-3 fatty acids from fish, as well as from supplements in capsule or liquid form). Foods high in unhealthy saturated fat include butter and cream, and foods high in healthy saturated fat include avocados and extra-virgin olive oil (in moderation).

3. Maximize high-quality lean protein. Foods high in lean protein include chicken breast (white meat) and fish (baked or grilled, not fried).

The first of these guidelines is the most important and the one that we will spend the most time discussing. Following these guidelines will help minimize the impact of AD; however, it is essential to understand *why* and *how* these and other strategies should be implemented. This book describes the rationale behind suggested dietary changes and offers clear guidance through a systematic dietary transformation to maximize brain health.

THE CUTTING-EDGE ALZHEIMER'S DIET APPROACH

It is only over the last decade that Alzheimer's disease has been recognized as a major public health crisis. Significant progress has been made in our understanding of how to fight this disease, but much more remains to be done. More recently, we have started scientifically testing the effects of dietary interventions on the development of AD. As modern science advances, we are beginning to make strides in our understanding of gut-brain interactions.

Because this information is so new, **most people are not yet aware of the influence that diet can have on Alzheimer's disease.** Until recently, even research scientists and medical doctors were unaware that dietary modification could improve brain function. To put this in perspective, it was not that long ago that both healthcare providers and the public at large first realized that cigarettes were bad for our lungs.

We used to give children pure morphine (a dangerous

According to nationwide surveys,

Doctors prefer
MILFORD
cigarettes over any other brand!

100 cardiologists were asked
"What brand of cigarettes do you smoke?"
The overwhelming choice was Milford!

SHOULDN'T YOU LISTEN TO YOUR DOCTOR?

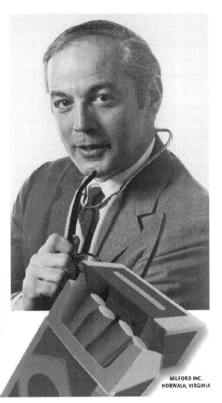

DR. ALFRED CONCENTURE smokes two packs of Milford cigarettes per day and recommends them to his patients. "The flavor of Milford cigarettes makes them the obvious choice."

DR. JONATHAN SMITH has been smoking Milford cigarettes for over thirty years. "Milford cigarettes are more mild than most other brands, so they are the obvious choice for me since I suffer from asthma."

DR. CHARLES SCHWECK is a loyal customer and spokesperson for Milford cigarettes. "I would not endorse any other brand but Milford. Other cigarettes contain chemicals, but Milford cigarettes are all natural."

MILFORD INC.
NORWALK, VIRGINIA

narcotic drug) in "soothing syrups," take diet pills containing tapeworms to lose weight, treat coughs with heroin, and soothe cuts by rubbing toxic mercury on them. And, of course, most people are familiar with the fact that until 1929, Coca Cola contained cocaine.

Just as our understanding of the negative effects of smoking cigarettes and illicit drug use has expanded, so has our knowledge of the negative health consequences of eating sugar-laden foods. We are now coming to realize just how detrimental excessive sugar intake can be to our bodies and brains. After reading this book, you will have knowledge that future generations will likely take for granted but few fully understand today.

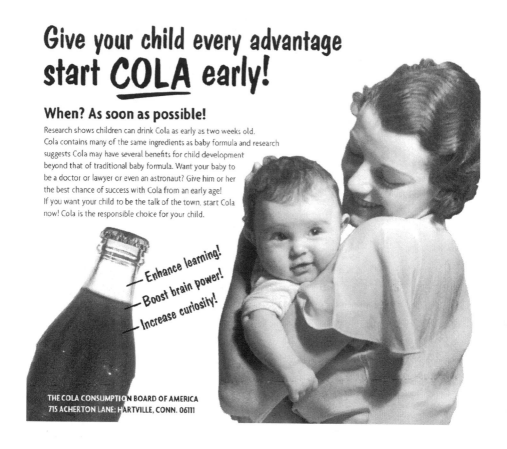

Give your child every advantage
start <u>COLA</u> early!

When? As soon as possible!

Research shows children can drink Cola as early as two weeks old. Cola contains many of the same ingredients as baby formula and research suggests Cola may have several benefits for child development beyond that of traditional baby formula. Want your baby to be a doctor or lawyer or even an astronaut? Give him or her the best chance of success with Cola from an early age! If you want your child to be the talk of the town, start Cola now! Cola is the responsible choice for your child.

Enhance learning!
Boost brain power!
Increase curiosity!

THE COLA CONSUMPTION BOARD OF AMERICA
715 ACHERTON LANE: HARTVILLE, CONN. 06111

CUTTING-EDGE RESEARCH

For any approach to any medical condition to be truly cutting-edge and effective, it must be based on the most recent scientific evidence—that is, data from high-quality scientific studies that have been rigorously conducted in the past several years. The recent surge in scientific research demonstrating that dietary interventions can improve thinking skills for AD patients (and potentially delay its onset for those at risk for developing AD) inspired the writing of this book. We describe this scientific evidence throughout and explain how this information can be applied in everyday life to improve regular dietary habits. Some brief examples are provided below, including for the condition mild cognitive impairment (MCI), which is a "pre" Alzheimer's disease condition discussed later in Chapter 1.

EXAMPLES OF CUTTING-EDGE RESEARCH ON NUTRITION AND ALZHEIMER'S DISEASE	
Vitamins	High-quality studies have shown that certain vitamins can improve memory in MCI patients and improve how certain FDA-approved drugs can work in patients with AD.
Omega-3 Fatty Acids	Recent scientific trials support the use of Omega-3 fatty acids from both eating certain types of fish and potentially taking specific supplements.
Medical Food	The medium-chain triglyceride caprylic acid is available as an FDA-regulated medical food for the clinical dietary management of AD.
Coffee	Laboratory studies have recently shown that specific amounts of certain types of coffee may have cognitive benefit.
Berries	Strong evidence supports regular intake of specific types of berries delays cognitive decline for over two years.
Cocoa Powder	MCI patients with regular intake of the strong antioxidants in cocoa powder had improved memory function, blood pressure, and insulin resistance.

If a patient or caregiver feels that he or she wants to do everything possible to fight this disease, as long as it is relatively safe, these proven dietary approaches will be an essential part of the management plan.

PART 2—WHO SHOULD BE READING THIS BOOK?

This book is useful for *anyone* who is concerned about his or her memory, regardless of whether he or she is at risk for, or has, Alzheimer's disease. Therefore, **anyone wishing to protect or improve his or her memory can benefit from reading this book!** Nonetheless, *The Alzheimer's Diet* is targeted toward people who want to learn how to utilize nutrition for the treatment or prevention of Alzheimer's disease and practical strategies for doing so.

One of the most common questions that we get asked about AD is "Am I at risk?" The answer is simple; since the number-one risk factor for AD is advancing age, then *everyone* is at risk of developing AD. However, the good news is that there is finally scientific evidence (more than 100 years after the first description of Alzheimer's as a disease) that we may be able to delay the onset of memory loss and treat AD through dietary changes.

At a recent *Alzheimer's Association International Conference*, researchers presented several new important findings showing that there are several risk factors that may increase a person's likelihood of developing AD. For example, having uncontrolled high blood pressure over many years can increase risk of cognitive decline and AD. A new mathematical model of risk factors for AD suggested that changing certain lifestyle-based behaviors (many of which are discussed in this book) by 25 percent could potentially prevent millions of AD cases throughout the world (Barnes and colleagues). The risk factors that contributed to AD included diabetes, mid-life high blood pressure, mid-life obesity, smoking, inadequate physical activity, low educational attainment, and depression. Modifying these risk factors may lower the risk of Alzheimer's disease and may also slow the progression or severity of the symptoms.

Another of the most common questions that we get asked about AD is "If I have a family history, am I more likely to develop Alzheimer's?" Before we answer this, let us clarify a few things. In general, Alzheimer's is a very common condition regardless of whether a person has a family member with the disease. In fact, **everyone's risk of developing AD increases over time because the number-one risk factor is advancing age**. That being said, there are specific genes that can be passed on from parents to children that may increase the likelihood of developing Alzheimer's disease. The good news is that only 6 percent of AD cases are caused by the types of genes that can lead to early-onset Alzheimer's disease. We will not get into technical detail here, but these genetic mutations include presenilin-1, presenilin-2, and amyloid precursor protein gene mutation. These genes may contribute to the development of AD in patients younger than age sixty, although many younger-onset patients do not end up having these genes.

There is another set of genes that are associated with older-age onset of AD, or late-onset Alzheimer's disease. The most well studied of these genes is called apolipoprotein epsilon-4 (or commonly referred to as APOE4 [or APOΕ-4]). Briefly, we get one copy of the APOE gene from our mother and another copy from our father. There are three types of these genes, APOE2, APOE3, and APOE4. If a person has one or more of the APOE4s, the risk of developing AD is increased. However, genetic testing for APOE is not currently recommended. Knowing whether a person has one or more copies of APOE4 does not necessarily help a physician predict if or when a patient will develop AD. Conversely, having one or more copies of APOE2 confers a reduced risk of developing AD.

We still have a long way to go before using genetic testing to help with the pre-symptomatic diagnosis of AD. For these reasons, Dr. Isaacson's does not recommend genetic testing on family members of Alzheimer's patients in his clinical practice. Instead, he suggests that all family members focus on a healthy lifestyle plan as detailed in this book.

KEY CONCEPT: Just because a person is getting older does not mean that he or she will necessarily develop Alzheimer's disease. However, some decline in memory function is normal with advancing age. Therefore, everyone can benefit from efforts to preserve and protect their memory.

Keep in mind that there are some changes in thinking skills that occur normally with age. This condition is called age-associated cognitive impairment. Symptoms may include intermittent memory loss, word-finding difficulties, and slowing of the speed of thinking. When cognitive changes are isolated to difficulties with memory, this condition is sometimes referred to as age-related memory loss.

We do not yet have all the answers about what would be considered the "normal" or expected cognitive changes that occur with age. Scientists also have much work to do to more accurately determine whether a person will develop AD instead of conditions like normal age-related memory loss. This is an area where active research is currently being conducted.

An extensive review of all of the risk factors for AD is beyond the scope of this book. However, influence of family history may depend on the number of first-degree relatives affected and if they were diagnosed early (before age sixty) or later in life. Earlier onset disease may be more likely to have a genetic component. The medical history of the patient is also important, and conditions such as Down's syndrome, heart disease, diabetes, metabolic syndrome, obesity, and head trauma have been associated with an increased risk of AD.

Again, much more scientific research is needed to clarify these points. There is a continually updated online database called the AlzRisk (AD Risk Factors) Epidemiology Database, available at: http://www.alzrisk.org/. See Appendix A in the back of the book for more information on this database, which highlights many of the areas currently being studied (e.g., alcohol use, hormone therapy, inflammatory biomarkers, and nutritional antioxidants).

In addition to the risk factors being studied above, the following is a short list of conditions that may also be associated with AD risk:

- High cholesterol (particularly LDL cholesterol)

- Diabetes

- Low thyroid function

- High blood pressure

- Head trauma associated with loss of consciousness (particularly in people with the APOE4 gene)

- Female gender (potentially related to longer lifespan)

- History of major depression (associated with or precedes AD)

- Elevated homocysteine (an inflammatory marker in the blood)

- Walking impairment

- Chronic renal failure

Some of the most important protective factors to reduce AD risk include:

- Greater educational attainment and mentally challenging occupations

- APOE2 genes (or alleles)

- Exercise (physical and mental)

- Lifelong musical activity

- And of course . . . diet! (e.g., low carb, low saturated fat, and rich in specific types of fish and berries)

We hope this book raises awareness of the importance of diet for optimal brain health. More and more frequently, new scientific studies are published verifying the relation of nutrition to memory loss and AD. This book is an effort to summarize these advances for those concerned about memory loss, those patients and caregivers currently fighting AD, and healthcare providers (like doctors and nurses) also on the "front lines" in the battle against this condition. While our health conditions are far from being under our total control, please help us in our efforts to spread the word on how diet can help to offset memory loss. Today, everyone can, and should, change their nutrition patterns to better protect their brains!

SECTION 1

FUNDAMENTAL INFORMATION

CHAPTER 1

What Is Alzheimer's Disease and How Can Diet Help?

Alzheimer's disease (AD) is a condition in which a person progressively loses his or her memory and thinking skills. Frequently, these cognitive changes are attributed to the normal aging process. However, as time goes on, short-term memory declines and the most common problems include loss of orientation (e.g., not knowing the date or directions), difficulty with communication (inability to find the correct words to say), changes in behavior, and impaired judgment.

Some examples of memory loss include continually losing things, like keys or a cell phone. Misplacing objects, forgetting appointments, and repeating the same things over and over again are also common symptoms, which may be related to memory and/or concentration problems that are often observed in AD. While it is common for people as they age to occasionally forget things (like names) and even misplace objects, usually people are able to remember the names later, as well as find the missing objects.

These examples of memory "loss" are quite different from the more significant memory complaints that progressively worsen in AD. For example, it can be normal to forget the name of an old acquaintance that you have not seen in a long time. Usually that name will be on the "tip of your tongue" and recalled later. This is an expected change that comes with aging. Also, with constant life distractions (like text messages and emails coming in on the cell phone, or children shouting in the background), it is common for people to forget things since they were not able to pay attention while they were happening. For more information on this topic, visit www .TheADplan.com/mediacenter.htm, and watch Dr. Isaacson and Amy Brightfield of *Woman's Day* magazine discuss the difference between routine forgetfulness and severe memory loss on the NBC *Today* Show with Kathie Lee and Hoda.

Interestingly, the first observable signs of AD may not actually be memory loss, but may instead be a depressed mood, a loss of interest in pleasurable activities, a change in

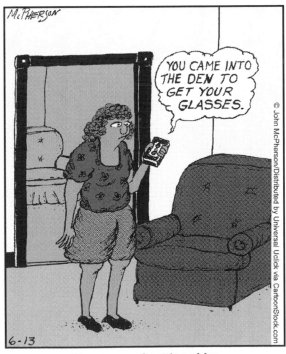

The agony of getting older.

personality, increasing anxiety, a change in sleep patterns, or even a loss or decrease in sense of smell. We are strong advocates for early diagnosis, so it is advisable for people to seek medical attention when symptoms first begin. A variety of specialists including primary care doctors (internist or family doctor), neurologists, geriatric psychiatrists, or geriatricians (specializing in the care of people age sixty-five and over) can be called upon to perform an evaluation.

KEY CONCEPT: The earlier doctors can diagnose AD, the earlier they can treat—and the earlier they can treat, the better the patient will do.

AD is the most common form of dementia, representing approximately two-thirds of all cases. The most recent statistics show that one out of seven people age seventy-one and over have dementia, and over 45 percent of individuals over the age of eighty-five have AD. According to the Alzheimer's Association 2012 statistics, there are over 5.4 million people in the United States with AD.

For the most part, the dietary strategies discussed in this book target specific biological abnormalities that both precede the onset, and occur throughout the duration, of Alzheimer's disease. Some strategies aim to reduce inflammation in the brain (e.g., omega-3 fatty acids), improve blood flow (via optimizing control of abnormal blood pressure, blood sugar, and cholesterol), reduce detrimental protein deposits (e.g., exercise), or give the brain more "fuel" to function (e.g., medical food, very low-carbohydrate diet).

AD is a very complex disease, and scientists still do not understand all of its intricacies. Most of the options discussed in this book have been shown to be effective, but how or why some of them work remains unclear. A good example of this is exercise. For years, clinicians recommended exercise for AD treatment and prevention because "it was good for you." This is not a very scientific answer. In the past, physicians theorized that exercise increased blood flow to the brain or released chemicals into the bloodstream that improved memory and thinking skills, but they lacked evidence supporting this theory. We now understand that regular exercise may help to increase blood flow to the brain and know more about which specific chemicals are released and how they make the brain function better. Recent data has shown that regular exercise maintains heart function, and that alone relates to a larger brain volume (which is related to IQ and memory function). More recently, scientists have discovered that exercise reduces the pathologic protein in the AD brain called amyloid (or beta-amyloid protein).

DEFINITION: **Beta-amyloid Protein**

A protein found in excess in the brains of patients with AD. This protein sticks together and forms plaques, or clumps, which may interfere with normal brain cell function.

A more detailed discussion of the neurobiology of AD and the mechanism of each intervention is beyond the scope of this book. Suffice it to say that, while we may not know exactly how some of these interventions work to improve symptoms or delay onset of AD, there is clinical and/or scientific evidence supporting their effectiveness.

ALZHEIMER'S DISEASE DIAGNOSIS

While this book focuses primarily on dietary strategies for the treatment and prevention of AD, we feel it is important to briefly review the two most commonly used diagnostic criteria for this disease. This is important since the ways that physicians diagnose AD have recently changed. For many years, physicians have used the criteria in the *Diagnostic and Statistical Manual of Mental Disorders* for diagnosing AD. These criteria are overall very good and are currently the most common criteria that are used; however, in the future this may change to the newer criteria described below.

In order to meet criteria for Alzheimer's disease, a person needs to have the onset of memory problems described earlier plus one or more of the following:

1. Problems with language or speaking skills ("aphasia")

2. Difficulty performing movements or tasks, such as combing hair, brushing teeth, or driving ("apraxia")

3. Difficulty recognizing objects like a remote control to the television or a pencil ("agnosia")

4. Impaired judgment or thinking skills for everyday activities ("executive function")

A diagnosis of Alzheimer's disease would be considered when these difficulties interfere with the normal activities of daily living, represent a decline from prior functioning, and occur with a gradual onset and a slowly progressive course that cannot be explained by any other non-brain disease (e.g., thyroid dysfunction, "pseudodementia" of depression).

The earliest stages of AD are most often referred to as "mild Alzheimer's disease." As the disease progresses, physicians may then call the disease "moderate AD" and, as it continues to progress, "severe AD." There is no clear consensus among physicians on when to use the terms "mild," "moderate," or "severe." Some physicians will use results of cognitive testing, and others will determine severity based on how the patient is functioning on an everyday basis.

In April 2011, new AD diagnostic criteria were published based on the recommendations of an expert panel convened by the National Institute on Aging and the Alzheimer's Association. These criteria include three "stages" of AD:

1. A diagnosis of *dementia due to Alzheimer's disease*

2. A diagnosis of *mild cognitive impairment (MCI) due to Alzheimer's disease*

3. A diagnosis of *"preclinical" Alzheimer's disease*

DEFINITION: **Mild Cognitive Impairment (MCI)**

Essentially a "pre-Alzheimer's" medical condition in which patients have about a 12 percent chance per year of developing AD. Patients may have problems with memory, language, thinking skills, or judgment, although these symptoms do not yet cause functional changes or other limitations in their daily lives.

These three classifications are helpful since they set the stage for future advances in AD by incorporating "biomarkers" in the diagnostic criteria. A biomarker is something that can be used to more accurately diagnose AD, like a blood test or a radiology study. Currently, there is no test available that can diagnose AD with 100 percent accuracy despite the fact that evidence of AD starts in the brain many years before clinical symptoms appear. We hope that early and completely accurate diagnosis will become possible, but this is still many years in the future. Eventually, we may be able to perform a simple test (e.g., blood, spinal fluid, brain scan) and then begin treatment many years before the onset of AD symptoms. In fact, for the first time in 2012, the FDA approved a brain-imaging test that may be able to help diagnose patients with cognitive impairment who are being evaluated for AD and other causes of memory loss and cognitive decline. It is important to note, however, that this technology has not yet led to wide-spread use since a "positive" scan does not 100 percent establish a diagnosis of AD as opposed to another cognitive disorder. In addition, the effectiveness of this scan

DR. ISAACSON:

In my clinical experience, and now based on the new criteria, patients with MCI may most commonly have "pre-Alzheimer's," or prodromal AD (at risk for developing AD). Patients in this category may derive benefit from a variety of interventions that may be best suited for use early in the onset of memory loss. There are several ongoing scientific research trials that are currently investigating this important area.

has not been established for predicting development of a specific type of dementia.

As mentioned in the new diagnostic criteria, mild cognitive impairment (MCI) is commonly characterized by changes in thinking skills that have been identified by a physician, but these changes have not yet impacted the patient's activities of daily living.

NORMAL BRAIN AGING VERSUS ALZHEIMER'S DISEASE

It is common for the brain to age over time, but as discussed earlier, not all of those changes are due to AD. For example, young children can much more easily learn a new language while they are growing up compared to a college student or older adult who is learning a new language for the first time. Research shows that older adults process information less efficiently than healthy young adults. This is likely due to the accumulation of damage to brain cells over time. Brain cells can be damaged for many reasons, most commonly due to risk factors affecting blood flow to the brain (e.g., high blood pressure). Brain cells can also be damaged from things like repeated head injury or concussions, for example. In fact, Dr. Isaacson cares for several retired football players who have sustained decade-long and repeated head trauma, which may increase the risk of cognitive decline, as well as AD.

Aging is also associated with an increased risk of damage to the blood vessels. Medical conditions like high cholesterol and diabetes can increase the chance of a damage to brain cells, which in turn can lead to a decline in memory function and thinking skills.

Scientists have a long way to go to fully understand the differences between normal or expected cognitive changes that occur with age versus brain changes due to common chronic medical problems (like untreated high blood pressure) versus AD.

One of the areas that researchers have focused on is beta-amyloid protein. This can accumulate in the brain of people with AD. While this is the characteristic pathologic finding in AD, evidence of amyloid has also been found in non-AD individuals at younger ages. In addition, up to one-third of normal individuals over the age of sixty-five have amyloid in their brain. While it is not known whether these people will definitely go on to develop AD, anything we can do to lower the amount of beta-amyloid in the brain (like exercise) may in the future be proven to protect both normal brain aging as well as AD.

The graph below demonstrates how the buildup of beta-amyloid occurs many years before the onset of the diagnosis of MCI and AD.

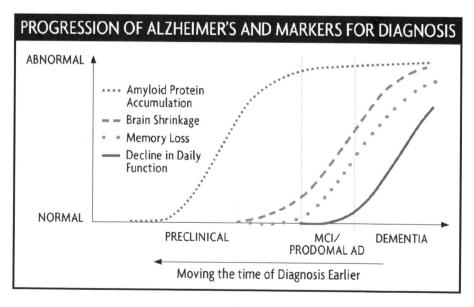

CHAPTER 2

The Alzheimer's Epidemic: Food Intake, the Brain, and the Carbohydrate Connection

The Alzheimer's epidemic may be the greatest public health crisis facing our world today. In addition to the over 5 million Americans with Alzheimer's disease (AD), millions more are affected throughout Canada, Europe, and the rest of the world. This explosion in the prevalence of Alzheimer's disease is in part due to the advancing age of our population. For example, in 2011, "baby boomers" in the United States first began to turn sixty-five. Given that the number-one risk factor for AD is advancing age, and the increasing age of the general population, **the number of AD cases is projected to more than triple by the year 2050!**

However, it is important to note that the advancing age of our population is not the sole factor in the prevalence of this disease. Many experts feel that the rise in AD cases is also due to other factors, such as the improved diagnostic techniques leading to more frequent diagnoses. This would suggest that the incidence of AD has been much higher than estimated in previous years, but we are just now able to see this (due to more sophisticated and/or sensitive testing).

Recent scientific evidence suggests that changes in dietary

and nutritional patterns may also be a causal factor in the rising number of AD cases. This is particularly true in the United States, throughout Europe, and other industrialized nations, where other nutrition-related epidemics (obesity and diabetes) have also increased in the past several decades. In the past twenty to thirty years, there have been dramatic increases in fast-food chains, processed foods, added sugars, portion sizes, and food intake. People are eating more sugar and fat, and fewer fruits and vegetables, than ever before. In addition to obesity and diabetes, these habits have also been associated with a higher risk of developing AD.

A variety of mechanisms have been proposed to relate why high dietary sugar (carbohydrate) intake causes insulin resistance, and subsequently how this can lead to the development of cognitive decline and AD. Common conditions like diabetes (also called diabetes mellitus, or type 2 diabetes) cause insulin resistance over time. This may lead to brain dysfunction (e.g., memory loss) and can also lead to age-related cognitive decline, mild cognitive impairment, and AD. Again, a discussion of causal mechanisms is beyond the scope of this book, but it is important to be aware of this connection.

DEFINITION: **Insulin Resistance**

A condition where the body does not respond properly or becomes "resistant" to the effect of insulin in lowering blood sugar levels.

Most people understand that excess sugar is "bad" when it comes to obesity and diabetes. But many are unaware of the long- and short-term effects of carbohydrates, particularly sugar, on brain function and memory. There are several different types and varieties of carbohydrates, and in terms of increasing the risk of AD, all carbohydrates are not the same. Incrementally reducing carbohydrate intake may decrease the likelihood of developing AD in the future. Moreover, a more significant reduction of carbohydrates may be necessary *after* a person develops AD, in order to have a therapeutic benefit. This is discussed further below and in Section 2.

FOOD INTAKE AND THE BRAIN

It is well known that the brain controls behavior, including decisions about which and how much food we eat. Until recently, however, the significant impact that the food we eat has on our brain function was largely overlooked.

What we eat affects the brain through different pathways. For example, some of the nutrients in the foods we eat can themselves directly affect the brain (since they can penetrate directly into the brain, by crossing what is referred to as the "blood-brain barrier"). Other times, the food we eat causes the release of certain chemicals (hormones) that enter and affect brain function. In this book, we focus on the long-term effect of dietary patterns on brain function, particularly memory. Although we emphasize making changes to last a lifetime, it is important to note that even short-term changes in dietary patterns can have a positive effect on memory and other health-related conditions.

YOU ARE WHAT YOU EAT!

Essentially, the food that we eat provides fuel for our brains.

Just like a car, low-quality fuel can lead to premature degradation (aging) of the engine and decreased performance. Conversely, high-quality fuel can actually clean out some of the "gunk" that builds up over time and improve engine performance. **The brain is like a finely tuned automobile engine that needs high-quality fuel to function at peak performance.**

Over a lifetime, low-quality fuel can be a major contributing factor to declining memory performance, or cognitive impairment. In subsequent chapters, we will discuss as clearly as possible the science behind this concept. For those who have not been providing high-quality fuel for their brains (which is most people in Westernized countries throughout the world), there is good news: it is not too late! We specialize in teaching people how to select the best fuel to have their brains firing on all cylinders.

That being said, we should take a moment to talk about expectations. We are not suggesting that following this diet will have every brain running like a Formula-1 race car fresh from production. As you probably already understand, there is no cure or magic bullet for Alzheimer's disease. So, while the information in this book can help anyone get the best performance out of his or her brain, dietary changes should not be the only therapeutic approach adopted. The brain is infinitely more complex than even the most high-performance car engine and more powerful than even the most advanced super computer. That being the case, we consider using the right fuel for the brain necessary, but not sufficient, for peak performance.

The strategies detailed in this book should be used as part of a multi-modal treatment and prevention approach. Details on this approach can be read online at websites like www .TherapyForMemory.org, and for the latest information and scientific research, read the blog on www.TheADplan.com/ blog. Also, updates are available on Facebook at www.Facebook.com/AlzheimersDisease or on Twitter at www.twitter .com/TheADplan.

Just like different car engines, different people have different biological limits to their memory function that cannot be overcome. This means that a person's genetic makeup (the genes or DNA that everyone gets as a combination from their mom and dad) will, at times, dictate the results of specific dietary changes on health outcomes. This is a field of study called nutrigenomics, which will be covered in Chapter 15.

The dietary strategies discussed in this book are a vital component of a comprehensive plan designed to maximize memory function. While no one single strategy will be able to stop someone from developing AD or cure AD symptoms once diagnosed, a combination of several of the scientifically-based dietary strategies outlined in this book will provide the highest chance for success.

CARBOHYDRATE INTAKE AND THE BRAIN

The role of sugar and carbohydrates is one of the most important concepts in the Alzheimer's Diet. Here we provide some background on this subject and later talk more about how it can be applied toward improving brain health. For

DR. ISAACSON:

My recent research has focused on the "real life" aspects of diet modification for AD. I have tried to determine optimal ways to address the challenges that my patients (and their family members and caregivers) have encountered. In one small pilot study, the first research question we aimed to answer was how often an individual was able to follow my dietary recommendations for a continuous 9-week period. The results? Less than 40 percent of the time. Better than zero but still a lot less than 100 percent.

Subsequent research by Dr. Ochner and me has yielded some very interesting results, which we most recently presented at the international Clinical Trials in Alzheimer's Disease conference in Monte Carlo, Monaco (October 29–31, 2012). Overall, this work has tried to address the following research questions:

1. What strategies may improve adherence to the Alzheimer's Diet detailed in this book?

2. What challenges can be addressed?

3. What methods of diet and nutrition education work best?

4. Can an online computerized database tool help patients and family members in the fight against AD?

Presented to the scientific community for the first time in Monte Carlo, this tool called the Alzheimer's disease—Nutrition Tracking System (AD-NTS) was designed to allow users to:

- Organize and understand dietary patterns related to brain health
- Record markers of progress before and after dietary change have been made
- Communicate this progress with treating physicians and healthcare providers.

We are extremely excited to now share this resource with the public, and encourage you to visit www.AlzheimersDiet.com to learn more and access the AD-NTS.

example, we encourage individuals to minimize carbohydrates called "simple sugars." Simple sugars include the type of sugar people put in their coffee (cane sugar), as well as more concentrated versions such as high fructose corn syrup (and corn syrup in general).

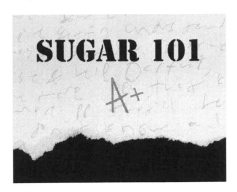

The Problem: Too much sugar over time is bad for the brain. It causes surges of insulin release in the body that over time may impair a person's ability to process sugar. In the brain, too much insulin leads to inflammation, which can promote the development and worsening of Alzheimer's disease.

The Solution: As Mom says, "Everything in moderation." When it comes to sugar, less is more, and substitute with sugar alternatives (e.g., Stevia) when possible. Learn about the different types of sugar, and how those with a high glycemic index may be the most harmful.

DEFINITION: **Insulin**

A hormone released by the body in response to sugar intake, and responsible for regulating blood sugar levels. High insulin levels are associated with inflammation in the brain.

Sugars can either be "added" or "naturally occurring." An added sugar is a sugar or syrup that is added to foods during processing or preparation. These do not include naturally occurring sugars such as fructose (in fruits) or lactose (in milk products). As mentioned, sugar is a form of carbohydrate, which is processed or metabolized by the body for energy. However, the body can only process a certain amount of carbohydrate to be used as fuel from any given meal. The leftover calories (not used for fuel) are stored as fat, which is not good for the body or brain.

An important part of the process is the body's production of insulin, which (among other things) regulates the amount of glucose in the blood. Blood glucose is the primary sugar that the body makes from the food in the diet. It is vital for proper body and brain functioning. However, too much or too little is problematic. Glucose is routinely carried through the bloodstream, and the cells in the body require insulin to utilize glucose. When the body is functioning properly, the amount of insulin produced is in tune with the amount of carbohydrate ingested. These concepts will be explained later in greater detail.

As we will continuously emphasize, **all carbohydrates are not created equal!** On the most basic level, carbohydrates can be classified as either simple or complex. Simple carbohydrates are easily and quickly metabolized by the body and cause a rapid spike in insulin levels. This is bad. What we commonly refer to as "table sugar" is actually a simple carbohydrate. Conversely, complex carbohydrates are not as easily metabolized by the body and cause a more gradual elevation of insulin levels. This is good. This relates to the "glycemic index" of food, which is an important term to understand.

DEFINITION: Glycemic Index

A classification proposed to quantify the relative blood glucose response to carbohydrate-containing foods (http://www.health.gov). It is a ranking on a scale from 0 to 100 for carbohydrates according to the extent to which they raise blood glucose levels and how much insulin is released by the body in response. In other words, for the carbohydrate that is eaten (e.g., cane sugar vs. white rice vs. whole wheat pasta), the glycemic index tells us how much insulin is released by the body in response to eating that food. Low-glycemic index foods produce a less pronounced increase in blood glucose and insulin levels, likely due to their slow metabolism, digestion, and/or absorption (good). High-glycemic index foods cause a more pronounced increase or "spike" in blood glucose and require more insulin to metabolize (bad).

LIMITING CARBOHYDRATES (ESPECIALLY THOSE WITH A HIGH-GLYCEMIC INDEX)

Common foods that are considered as high-glycemic carbohydrates include white bread, white rice, most sodas (due to the main ingredient of high-fructose corn syrup), cakes, and cookies. Common carbohydrate foods that are considered low on the glycemic scale include most fruits and vegetables, nuts, and beans. Food items like rye and whole-wheat bread, oat bran, and basmati rice would fall in the medium category of glycemic index. Refer to Appendix D for a more extensive list of brain-healthy options, including those with a low-glycemic index.

Recent research findings help illustrate why we advocate for the specific dietary change of carbohydrate restriction in people at risk for developing AD and in those who have already been diagnosed. Here we turn to randomized trials, which are considered high-quality research and are often necessary to prove or disprove the effectiveness of an intervention for a particular disease. In 2011, researchers showed that AD patients, who adhere to a low carbohydrate and low saturated fat diet, demonstrate significant improvement in memory performance (Craft). Another study showed that patients with MCI, or "pre-Alzheimer's," who adhere to a very low carbohydrate diet also show improved memory function (Krikorian 2010). These two are just a sampling of the research.

THE NOT-SO-SWEET TRUTH

Earlier in 2012, Dr. Sanjay Gupta (CNN medical correspondent) interviewed several leading scientists about the potential dangers of sugar. Visit http://www.cbsnews.com/8301-18560_162-57407294/is-sugar-toxic/ to watch the video and read more. Below, Dr. Ochner explains the evidence shown in this video, and how it relates to the philosophy behind the Alzheimer's Diet.

Why is too much sugar bad for your brain? This is another area where more research is needed, but we will discuss the most common theories about the association between sugar intake, memory function, and AD. What we do know for sure is that there is a connection between exces-

DR. OCHNER:

In addition to appointments at Columbia University and the NY Obesity Nutrition Research Center, I serve as an Associate Research Scientist at the Oregon Research Institute, where I collaborate with my colleague Dr. Eric Stice. Eric, who is featured in this video putting Dr. Sanjay Gupta in an fMRI scanner, is a world-leading expert on how the brain both controls and reacts to the intake of sugary foods. In this video, Eric discusses how recent brain-imaging studies show that the brain's reaction to ingesting sugar and drugs of abuse, such as cocaine, are strikingly similar.

sive sugar intake and memory impairment. The kicker is that the massive increases in sugar intake all around the world, and potential development of "sugar addiction," may have been inadvertently fueled by government programs designed to reduce the very same harmful effects caused by excessive sugar intake (e.g., heart disease).

The truth is that the amount of sugar the average person spoons out and adds to foods (aside from desserts) is small relative to the amount of sugar consumed unknowingly through regular foods and beverages. As discussed later, in the 1970s dietary fat was thought to be the main cause of heart disease. The government created regulations to lower the concentration of saturated fats in available foods, which was successful. However, the rate of heart disease increased! It is not that scientists at the time were wrong *per se*, just that we did not yet realize how adaptable our bodies were or how strong the evolutionary drive to store energy as fat was.

In order to try to maintain palatability (good taste), saturated fats were replaced with large quantities of sugar and/or high-fructose corn syrup (nutritionally considered the same thing, though some researchers suggest that high-fructose corn syrup may be worse for your brain than regular sugar). Most people, and even most scientists, believed that this was a fair trade for fat reduction. At the time, scientists believed that fat, especially saturated fat, was the worst thing a person could eat. Even ten years ago, most nutrition experts probably still would have agreed with this. However, what we are now discovering is that **sugar is converted to fat and stored in the body potentially even easier than the fat contained in the foods we eat!**

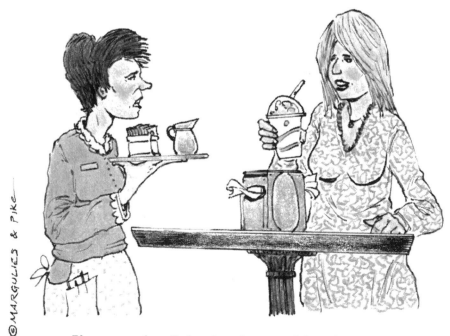

I'm a purist. I don't take anything in my Vanilla Mocha Dulce Latte.

Our sugar obsession has progressed to the point that the average American now consumes an astounding 130 *pounds* of sugar every year! Combine that with more restaurant eating and massive increases in portion sizes over the last thirty years, and this may be a driving factor behind the increase in AD in certain populations.

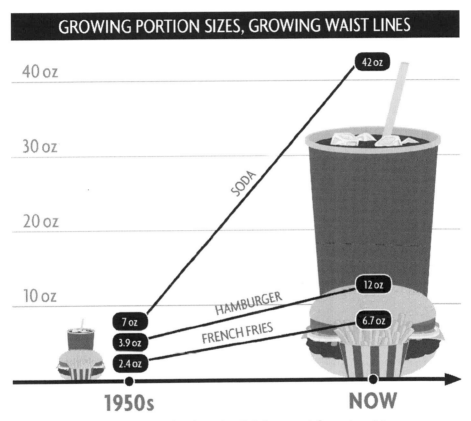

GROWING PORTION SIZES, GROWING WAIST LINES

40 oz

30 oz

20 oz

10 oz

42 oz

SODA

12 oz

7 oz

HAMBURGER

6.7 oz

3.9 oz

FRENCH FRIES

2.4 oz

1950s

NOW

Based on data on file from the CDC, for more information visit
http://makinghealtheasier.org/newabnormal

To elaborate on the graphic above, portion sizes have been steadily increasing over the last several decades. It is no surprise that the obesity epidemic has followed, along with increases in the amount of food that we eat. The average restaurant meal today is more than *four times* larger than it was in the 1950s. In addition, adults are on average *26 pounds* heavier than they were fifty years ago. There are several things we can do to eat healthier, like ordering the smaller meals on the menu, splitting a meal with a friend, or eating half and taking the rest home.

We know that excessive sugar intake increases a person's chances of developing both type-2 diabetes and AD, that diabetes is a risk factor for developing AD, and that controlling sugar intake is beneficial for both diabetes and AD. Therefore, a good diabetic diet is also a good brain diet. Thus, some of the concepts in the Alzheimer's Diet are based on those incorporated by patients with diabetes to control blood sugar. However, we also incorporate several other concepts that will help to maximize the brain health of your diet.

CHAPTER 3

When to Begin Diet Modification in the Fight Against Alzheimer's Disease

There is no time like the present to start making healthier dietary choices! However, the effect of diet on the overall health of the body starts much earlier—in the womb! Research has shown that the food a pregnant mother eats during pregnancy has an effect on future medical conditions and control of weight of the child. For example, one study in animals by Sinclair and colleagues showed that when mothers did not take in enough B vitamins (like folic acid and B12), the offspring was later at an increased risk of high blood pressure, fat accumulation, and insulin resistance (*Proceedings of the National Academy of Sciences*, 2007). Now of course, we are not animals, but this study and others like it shows that our future health is partially dependent on our mother's dietary habits. Making brain-healthy dietary choices will help to counteract the negative effects that aging and other medical conditions may have on the brain.

THE EFFECT OF AGING ON BRAIN FUNCTION

As we age, there are some changes in cognition that routinely occur. The severity of these changes can depend on a variety of genetic and environmental risk factors over one's lifespan. These risk factors may lead to several different causes of cognitive decline (e.g., Alzheimer's disease, age-associated cognitive decline). Conversely, there are several protective factors that may slow down brain aging. For example, the highest HDL cholesterol (high-density lipoprotein or "good" cholesterol) levels are associated with the most preserved thinking skills in individuals over 100 years old. In fact, there are several lifestyle factors (e.g., amounts of exercise and stress) and several medical conditions (e.g., vascular risk factors, metabolic syndrome, inflammation) that may positively or negatively relate to changes in thinking skills and memory.

As mentioned, healthy young adults are able to process information in their brain more efficiently (faster) than older adults with evidence of vascular damage. Several models have been proposed that help us understand the variety of factors that affect memory and cognition. One study called the Northern Manhattan Study (Dr. Sacco and colleagues) has been researching environmental and genetic aspects of age-related cognitive changes, in which patients have been followed for nearly twenty years. Based on this research, "successful" cognitive aging occurred in approximately 30 percent of patients. One way to help determine which patients will age successfully or have cognitive decline over time is by using a Global Vascular Risk Score. This score was developed as part of this study and takes into consideration markers such as obesity, blood pressure, exercise, and alcohol consumption. Many of these risk factors not only contributed to vascular damage in the brain, but also shrinkage of the brain and the progression and/or onset of Alzheimer's disease. Using a combination of these factors, an online calculator has been developed to provide an estimate of risk of future health issues. Visit http://neurology.med.miami.edu/gvr/gvr.htm for more information (website is for research purposes only and does not provide medical advice).

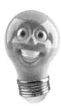 **KEY CONCEPT:** While the discussion in this book focuses on strategies for avoiding or delaying the onset of AD through diet and nutrition, several of these suggestions may help to delay the onset of other causes of cognitive decline as well.

There is often considerable disagreement over defining the "normal" (expected) cognitive changes that occur with age. We still have much to learn about the differences between Alzheimer's disease versus "normal" age-related cognitive changes versus other types of dementia. Both young and older individuals use complex brain networks (also called neural networks) that help to recall and remember things. The pathologic beta-amyloid protein that accumulates in the brain of AD patients may be responsible for memory dysfunction (perhaps less likely) or may occur as a result of another process that causes the dysfunction.

We also know that having a high level of "cognitive reserve" may improve outcomes when a cognitive disorder occurs in later life.

DEFINITION: **Cognitive Reserve**

The brain's "resistance" to memory loss and cognitive decline. This back-up system is based on how well the brain was able to function in earlier years. In other words, cognitive reserve refers to the brain's ability to manage the aging process with increasing damage, while still functioning as best as it can (through more well-developed brain networks and/or alternative cognitive strategies). Childhood cognition, educational attainment, and adult occupation all contribute to a person's cognitive reserve.

Building this reserve, or "backup," begins at birth, accelerates during schooling, and continues throughout young and mid-adult life. It seems that a high cognitive reserve offers some degree of protection against the severity of cognitive decline.

The build up of beta-amyloid may not be the answer here, and there is some data that contradicts the comments above. Another study led by Dr. Claudia Kawas at the University of California at Irvine is called the "90 plus study," which looks at individuals ninety years of age and older (with an average age of ninety-six!). In 2010, Kawas and colleagues published that, on average, one-third of the individuals in this study had dementia, one-third had cognitive impairment without dementia, and one-third were normal. When they looked at the brains of the participants of this study, nearly 50 percent of the patients had amyloid in their brain. However, many of these individuals were cognitively normal. Overall, it seems that having a high cognitive reserve may in fact allow a brain to function better longer, even in the presence of amyloid buildup.

In the 90 plus study, determinants of successful aging in normal individuals over the age of ninety were related to several factors including oxygenation, physical performance (hand grip, speed of walking), and blood pressure. It is not clear whether being on blood pressure medications was the cause of better cognition, or if having higher blood pressure increased blood flow to the brain.

When a blood pressure is taken, it is commonly reported as two numbers, for example, "130 over 70," or 130/70. The "top" number represents the systolic pressure and the "bottom" number represents the diastolic pressure. While some studies have shown diastolic blood pressure may be more relevant, other studies have found the opposite.

Based on significant research, better control of blood pressure may be a way to delay brain aging and preserve memory function for the future. Therefore, understanding and keeping track of blood pressure readings over time is important. Tracking forms are available at the back of the book and in the online AD-NTS at www.TheAlzheimers Diet.com.

The take-home point of this chapter is that the earlier

people begin adopting a healthy diet, thus offsetting certain risk factors (high blood pressure), the better chance they will have at revitalizing or saving their brain!

CHAPTER 4

Costs of Brain-Healthy versus Unhealthy Choices

Earlier, we discussed how the food that we eat is fuel for our brains and how the quality of fuel can have a significant impact on brain and memory function. In this chapter, we discuss some of the ways low-quality fuel may have a negative impact on the body and brain, as well as how high-quality fuel may have a positive impact. In addition, we will also cover some of the practical aspects about food selection, specifically how to make cost-effective brain-healthy food choices.

SHORT- AND LONG-TERM EFFECTS OF EATING SUBOPTIMAL FOODS

Eating certain types of foods, particularly refined or "simple" carbohydrates, causes blood sugar to spike. As described earlier, carbohydrates can be characterized in terms of glycemic index, meaning how much they raise blood sugar levels. Total carbohydrate intake may also be characterized by the glycemic load, which differs from index (in that it also takes into account the actual *amount* of carbohydrate delivered by the particular food or foods).

DEFINITION: Glycemic Load

Glycemic load is based on the glycemic index. It takes into account how much each gram of carbohydrate in the food raises blood glucose levels (glycemic index) *as well as how much carbohydrate* is contained in particular foods.

For example, one slice of white bread has a higher glycemic *index* than one slice of rye bread. However, one slice of white bread has a lower glycemic *load* than two slices of rye bread. Similarly, brown rice and quinoa (pronounced *keen-wah*) have a lower glycemic *index* than white rice. However, a half cup of white rice has a lower glycemic *load* than a full cup of brown rice or quinoa. Therefore, **it is not just the glycemic index of food that is important, but the total amount of carbohydrate received from the food (glycemic load)**. For examples of brain-healthy options, including those with a low-glycemic load, see Appendix D in the back of the book.

After eating a meal with a high-glycemic load, a person may feel "good" immediately, but a sharp spike in blood sugar means a sharp decline (i.e., "crash") is soon to follow. This crash in blood sugar means a crash in energy as well, with no fuel left to run the body. It is as if someone wanted to heat his or her house with a wood-burning stove. Eating foods characterized with a high-glycemic load is like trying to keep the fire going by tossing in only paper and kindling. This "fuel" will very quickly burn up in a blustery flame and leave nothing to keep the fire going.

Conversely, eating foods characterized by a low-glycemic

load that are low in saturated fat and contain protein is like using perfectly seasoned logs instead of paper. They burn true every time, keeping the temperature steadily warm and providing ideal fuel for hours.

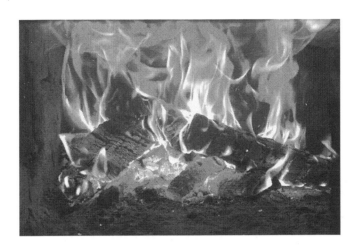

Foods with a low-glycemic load take longer to be processed (digested) and distributed throughout the blood-stream. This allows energy use to be maximized while minimizing the amount that is stored as fat. Low-glycemic foods do not cause a sudden violent spike, and subsequent crash, in blood sugar. How do these fluctuations cause negative effects over time in the brain? The answer lies in the relation to insulin, which when secreted in high amounts may cause damaging brain inflammation, with subsequent accelerated brain aging.

The costs of making unhealthy food choices over a long period of time are significant. In fact, most of the chronic diseases that our society faces were either caused or worsened by nutrition patterns over time (e.g., diabetes, high blood pressure, high cholesterol, and cognitive impairment, specifically AD). Conversely, there are several health benefits of low-glycemic eating. Typically, low-glycemic foods contain more nutrients since fruits and vegetables are more often utilized as a carbohydrate source. In addition, individuals can actually eat greater amounts of food since components are lower in energy density. Lower glycemic eating also has the potential to lead to weight loss in overweight and obese individuals, and improve blood sugar control in insulin resistant and diabetic individuals. Finally, low-glycemic foods may have increased amounts of fiber (often helping to slow the rate of digestion), which may decrease feelings of hunger.

Aside from minimizing the negative health effects of insulin, there are several theories as to why minimizing carbohydrates may be useful when it comes to brain function. One theory relates to the production of ketone bodies, which can be used as an alternative fuel source for the brain and may help reduce oxidative damage inside brain cells (in mitochondria).

DEFINITION: **Ketone Bodies**

Compounds produced when certain fats are metabolized (broken down) by the liver. Ketone bodies are the only other compound besides glucose that the brain can use for fuel.

Researchers have shown that a person with AD has a decreased ability to use glucose (sugar) as a fuel in the brain. Since the only alternative energy source aside from glucose that the brain can use for fuel is ketone bodies, this therapeutic target has been an area of active investigation. Chapters 14 and 23 will go into greater detail about this area.

Another theory on the benefits of minimizing carbo-hydrate intake is based on the role of insulin, especially as it relates to consumption of high-glycemic index carbohydrates. Insulin's effects on aging of the brain have been studied in detail. Insulin regulation affects longevity in every known animal species and plays a role in brain aging (Barbieri, 2003). Insulin attaches to the primary memory center in the brain (hippocampus), where it also has a direct influence on brain chemistry (Apelt, 2001).

Insulin resistance is a condition in which insulin cannot carry out its usual activities. Insulin resistance is associated with a variety of medical conditions, including obesity, high blood pressure, and high cholesterol. In addition, insulin and beta-amyloid (the pathologic protein found in the brain of patients with AD) are related. Studies have shown that insulin raises beta-amyloid in adults over age seventy and also increases brain inflammation (Watson, 2003).

This explanation only scratches the surface at understand-ing the interaction between insulin, inflammation, and the development of AD. However, even a basic understanding of the negative effects of insulin should explain why carbo-hydrate reduction is a sensible idea for brain protection. Reducing carbohydrates in the diet is easier said than done; however, making smarter carbohydrate choices is possible through education and discipline.

MONETARY COSTS

The amount of money we spend on food depends on a variety of factors, including actual cost of specific food ingredients, food handling (whether foods are "organic" or "processed," for example), preparation time, and where it is purchased. The largest monetary factor, however, is whether food is prepared and consumed inside or outside the home (home cooked vs. from a restaurant). The high cost of dining out and takeout is one reason we strongly encourage individuals adopting a brain-healthy diet to prepare their meals at home.

Organic food is generally more expensive, but the quality control may also be higher. Thus, specialty food markets tend to charge more but provide generally higher quality items. Whether having organic products is worth the additional cost is up to each individual. **Remember, however, that just because a food is organic does not necessarily mean that it is healthy.** In fact, *organic* has nothing to do with the macronutrient content of the food; it just means that the food is not processed. Overall, we recommend focusing more on the nutritional goals and guidelines presented in this book, rather than on specifically choosing organic foods. However, if financial means allow a person to purchase organic brain-healthy food, we encourage them to do so.

DEFINITION: Organic Food

Food that is certified to be produced by certain standards (e.g., handling, storage, production) and ingredients are free from prohibited substances (e.g., synthetic pesticides, chemical fertilizers) and are not genetically modified. In the United States, production is managed via the Organic Foods Production Act (OFPA), which integrates cultural, biological, and mechanical methods that foster "cycling of resources, promote ecological balance, and conserve biodiversity."

DEFINITION: Processed Foods

Any food that has been altered, or changed, from its natural state. This may occur due to convenience (e.g., storage or packaging) or for safety reasons (e.g., "pasteurization" of milk and orange juice, which is a process to kill bacteria). Not all processed foods are "bad" *per se,* but often when foods are canned, frozen, or dehydrated, some of the "good" nutrients are lost, and some "bad" ingredients are added.

There are plenty of brain-healthy foods at regular or even discount warehouse food stores, but care should be taken to avoid the abundance of processed foods in their aisles. Processed foods may have specific additives that render a food less healthy. For example, many canned foods have large amounts of added salt, which is not advisable for people with high blood pressure and other medical conditions. Processed meats have been linked to higher rates of certain types of cancers, like colon cancer. Individually packaged snacks like cookies and candies may have high amounts of sugar, calories, salt, and fat.

That said, anyone following the Alzheimer's Diet should anticipate an increase in food expenses during the initial 9-Week Diet Plan. This is, in part, due to the need to revamp the home food environment and partly due to the fact that it will take people some time to become familiar with more brain-healthy food options and where to find them at low cost. We think of this as one of the best investments anyone can make. After the 9-week period, however, food expenses should return to normal with a little planning.

CHAPTER 5

Body Weight and Alzheimer's Disease

How is obesity related to memory and thinking skills? Before we begin this discussion, there is a metric called the body-mass index (BMI) with which all health-conscious people should be familiar: BMI is a fairly straightforward way to measure a person's weight adjusted for height (measured in kg/m2 or weight in kilograms divided by height in meters squared). To have your BMI automatically calculated for you (as well as tracked over the course of the diet plan), go to the AD-NTS and enter your weight and height.

DEFINITION: **Body-Mass Index (BMI)**

A number calculated using weight and height. BMI can be used as a general to screen for weight categories that may lead to health problems. However, it does not directly measure a person's body fat.

Having a higher BMI and waist-to-hip ratio is linked to decreased size of the memory centers in the brain (hippocampus) later in life. Also, having high central adiposity (also known as a big stomach or "beer belly") increases risk of cognitive impairment (Whitmer and Yaffe, *Neurology* 2008).

To learn more about and calculate BMI, visit the Centers for Disease Control website (http://www.cdc.gov/healthy weight/assessing/bmi/). The table below details the four weight status categories paired with calculated BMI ranges.

BMI	WEIGHT STATUS
Below 18.5	Underweight
18.5—24.9	Normal
25.0—29.9	Overweight
30.0 and Above	Obese

A number of studies report an inverse relationship between body weight (particularly body fat) and memory function. This suggests that **more body fat is associated with worse memory function**. Although the effect of being overweight (BMI 25–29.9) on risk for developing AD is not as clear, the vast majority of evidence suggests a strong connection between obesity (BMI ≥ 30) and AD. For example, a large study, the findings of which were published in the journal *Current Alzheimer's Research*, followed over 10,000 men and women ages forty to forty-five for an average of thirty-six years, and found that **obese individuals were more than three times as likely to develop AD** relative to normal weight (BMI 18.5–24.9) individuals (Whitmer and colleagues, 2007).

Scientists are not exactly sure how being obese increases risk for developing AD so significantly. We know that obesity leads to vascular disease, impaired insulin responsiveness, and defective glucose metabolism. Therefore, based on research published in the *American Journal of Alzheimer's Disease & Other Dementias*, the negative effect of obesity may, at least in part, be due to vascular defects, impaired insulin metabolism, and/or a defect in glucose transport mechanisms in the brain (Naderali and colleagues, 2009). An in-depth discussion of these potential mechanisms is beyond the scope of this book, but the overall message here is that obesity and memory loss are related, and a diet to help one will likely help the other as well.

METABOLIC SYNDROME

Another common condition related to obesity is metabolic syndrome. This syndrome is a constellation of vascular risk factors that includes increased waist circumference, low HDL cholesterol, high triglycerides, high blood pressure, and abnormally elevated fasting blood glucose. Metabolic syndrome and obesity are both associated with accelerated cognitive aging, especially among those individuals with other medical illnesses that cause inflammation in the body.

All this being said, there is good news for those who are overweight. Research suggests that following the dietary suggestions in this book will likely lead to weight loss in addition to improvements in memory. In fact, the dietary changes described here may create a reciprocal benefit, since weight loss in obese individuals may have its own positive impact on memory function. However, weight loss *per se* is not a goal of the dietary strategies in this book.

A diet book that does not focus on weight loss may seem strange to some people. In fact, as a nutrition expert, it felt a little strange for Dr. Ochner to write and edit these words.

However, there are many kinds of diets, several of which do not focus on weight loss. Bodybuilders often follow diets tailored for weight gain. Athletes follow particular diets to maximize the performance of key muscles or physiological systems (e.g., the cardiovascular system). Other diets are tailored for particular conditions such as lactose intolerance, irritable bowel syndrome, celiac disease (gluten intolerance), and Crohn's disease (see www.MedicalNutritionFacts.com for some more examples). The diet outlined in this book is tailored for memory loss prevention and treatment, as part of a comprehensive management system for AD. However, as we said before, *anyone* concerned about memory loss may benefit by following these suggestions over a period of time. Thus, we prefer to think of this diet as one developed for "mental athletes" of all sizes and abilities, designed to maximize the performance of the brain.

CHAPTER 6

Meal Replacements in the Fight Against Alzheimer's Disease

Meal replacements represent an extremely useful dietary tool. The primary benefit is increased control and structure over eating. Completely controlling one's diet is not easy. If it were, we would likely not have the obesity epidemic we have. Particularly when beginning a dict plan, it will take time, effort, and likely some extra money to change eating habits, especially when a person has been following the traditional American diet throughout his or her life. Thus, replacing a meal with a pre-formulated meal replacement such as a nutrition bar or shake will help in a number of ways. These include:

- *Structure:* Increased dietary structure makes it much more likely that people will be able to stick to their planned diet.

- *Expense:* Meal replacements tend to be cheaper than purchasing a meal, even from most fast food restaurants.

- *Effort:* No meal could be easier to prepare than peeling back a wrapper or unscrewing a bottle cap. Not only does it save the effort that would be put forth to cook or purchase restaurant food, but there is no need to worry about the ingredients or preparation method or hidden carbs or saturated fat or . . . anything.

- *Time:* Many people cite time as a major barrier to eating healthy since it is faster to pick up a value meal from a local fast food restaurant than it is to cook a meal (which may or may not actually be true). Consuming one meal replacement per day eliminates 33 percent of food preparation (or purchasing) time.

- *Habit:* With the increased dietary structure provided by meal replacements comes the formation of healthier eating habits. People who smoke cigarettes, twirl their hair, crack their knuckles, or watch too much TV know that bad habits are hard to break. The good news, however, is that good habits tend to perpetuate once we get used to doing them.

- *Body Weight:* Meal replacements can not only provide the ideal fuel for your mind but also help with weight control.

No matter what, you will be receiving optimum nutrition for at least one of your three major meals. No muss, no fuss, just ideal nutrition. These reasons make diets that include meal replacements among the most effective diets available, regardless of your dietary goals (e.g., memory, weight loss, muscle building, etc.).

WHAT TO LOOK FOR IN A BRAIN-HEALTHY MEAL REPLACEMENT

The following are general guidelines to look for on the nutrition label when choosing a brain-healthy meal replacement.

As you will come to notice, there are very few, if any, meal replacements currently available that are highly optimized for brain nutrition.

OPTIMAL BRAIN-HEALTHY MEAL REPLACEMENT	
Total Fat	Approx. 5–7 grams (necessary for absorption of some vitamins, like D)
Saturated Fat	Less than or equal to 3 grams
Carbohydrate **Sugar**	10–20 grams is good; less than 10 grams is great less than 10 grams
Protein	1 gram of protein per every 10 calories
Vitamins	Look for Folic Acid, B6, B12, and D
Fiber	2–5 grams, more is better

CHAPTER 7

Vitamins & Dietary Supplements in Prevention and Treatment

R ecently, there has been significant research on the use of vitamin supplementation to prevent or delay the onset of AD. Additional studies have examined whether adding certain vitamins to the treatment regimen of patients with AD may also be beneficial. Certain vitamins have been shown to be beneficial for prevention and/or treatment, and these interventions typically have a favorable risk-benefit ratio, meaning they are generally safe.

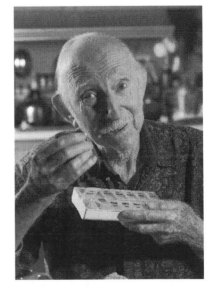

As an overview, vitamins fall under two separate categories: water soluble and fat soluble. Water-soluble vitamins (B and C) can be absorbed quickly and excess will be eliminated in the urine. Because of this quick absorption and elimination, water-soluble vitamins need continual replacement in the body. Fat-soluble vitamins (A, D and E), on the other hand, are stored in the liver and fatty tissue, and absorbed more slowly into the body.

Ideally, if one eats a healthy balanced diet, the Recommended Daily Allowance (RDA) of the essential vitamins should be mostly met via the foods that are eaten. The United States Department of Agriculture (USDA) agrees with this statement that nutritional needs should be met by eating a variety of foods as outlined in the Dietary Guidelines for Americans (most recently updated in 2011, for more information visit: http://www.cnpp.usda.gov/DGAs2010-PolicyDocument.htm).

DEFINITION: **Recommended Daily Allowance (RDA)**

The amounts of nutrients and calories an individual is recommended to consume each day. This includes amounts of vitamins and minerals, as recommended by the Food and Nutrition Board of the National Research Council.

As discussed in Chapter 3, when foods are processed, they are changed from their natural state and may lose part of their nutritional value. These processed foods can then be enriched with lost nutrients (e.g., vitamins). The USDA states that, in some cases, vitamin and mineral supplements (or fortified foods) may be useful for providing nutrients that may otherwise be eaten in less than the recommended amounts. Fortified foods have additional nutrients added in addition to the nutrients that occur naturally (non-processed foods).

DEFINITION: Enriched vs. Fortified

Enriched refers to the replacement of lost nutrients after processing. This includes the vitamins folic acid, iron, niacin, riboflavin, and thiamine, often necessary to meet FDA standards. When making food choices, enriched foods indicate that the food has been processed, thereby losing nutrients. Avoid this type of processed food when possible, and preferentially choose fresh or raw food, either with or without fortified nutrients.

Fortified refers to nutrients that are added to the food, in addition to the nutrients that were in the food originally. However, this does not necessarily make them a healthier option relative to fresh foods.

If a person is already eating the recommended amount of nutrients, they may not need to take supplements or select fortified foods since there may not be additional health benefits. However, when it comes to AD treatment and prevention, the studies described below involved taking additional vitamin supplements in pill form. These studies compared patients taking these vitamins with patients taking a placebo (or empty pill without any vitamins). When it comes to both AD treatment and prevention, it remains unclear whether a balanced diet can provide enough of these specific vitamins without additional supplementation in pill form.

So how can a person know whether or not they need to take vitamins in pill form in addition to a balanced diet? A thorough discussion with one's treating physician is advised, and reviewing the nutrition.gov and usda.gov websites can also be quite helpful (visit http://www.nutrition.gov/dietary-supplements/questions-ask-taking-vitamin-and-mineral-supplements, or http://fnic.nal.usda.gov/food-composition/individual-macronutrients-phytonutrients-vitamins-minerals for more information). In addition, the nutritional information obtained as part of the 9-Week Diet Plan will provide detailed information about a number of important vitamins and minerals, as well as the RDAs of each.

The USDA Dietary Guidelines for Americans makes specific recommendations for vitamin supplementation in certain groups of people. For example, many women of childbearing age (who may become pregnant) and those who are pregnant should eat foods rich in the B vitamin folic acid, in addition to eating fortified foods and/or supplements. Other USDA recommendations include:

- People over the age of fifty should consume vitamin B12 via supplements (pill form) or from fortified foods. This is due to the fact that older adults frequently have a reduced ability to absorb vitamin B12 from foods, and the type of vitamin B12 used in supplements and fortified foods is much more easily absorbed.

- Older adults, people with insufficient exposure to sunlight, and those with dark skin should consume extra vitamin D in supplement form or from fortified foods.

Remember that vitamin and mineral supplements are not a replacement for a healthy, balanced diet. Foods rich in vitamins and minerals also provide hundreds of naturally occurring substances that can help protect overall and most especially brain health.

VITAMINS FOR AD TREATMENT AND PREVENTION

Many physicians advocate for taking a multivitamin at least several times each week. Dr. Isaacson also suggests that his patients consider taking folic acid (1 mg total per day), B6, B12, and vitamin D3 (1,000–2,000 IU per day or more). As with all considerations, any supplement or vitamin must be taken with the approval and supervision of the treating physician (e.g., blood tests may need to be monitored).

Ensuring adequate intake of vitamins B and D via diet is essential, but many clinicians feel that patients may derive additional benefit when supplementing vitamin intake in pill form as well.

Studies have shown that a significant proportion of people are deficient in vitamin D, and that supplementation may be beneficial for brain protection. As such, in addition to adding 1,000–2,000 IU (or more) of vitamin D3 in pill form, this can be combined with at least 10–15 minutes of sunlight per day. The optimal dose of vitamin D3 is still unknown. Due to this uncertainty (e.g., dose, whether or not a blood level should be drawn), the decision to take vitamins and in what amounts should always be discussed with and approved by a person's primary-care physician.

A recent study by de Jager and colleagues (*International Journal of Geriatric Psychiatry*, 2011) studied the effect of B vitamins on cognitive functioning and clinical decline. B vitamins are known to lower a biomarker in the blood called homocysteine, which has also been found to be a potential risk factor for AD. In this double-blind study, MCI patients (ages seventy and above) with high homocysteine levels who received 0.8 mg of folic acid, 0.5 mg of vitamin B12, and 20 mg of vitamin B6 each day show improved cognitive test scores on a variety of commonly performed tests. These included the Mini Mental State Examination (scored on a 0 to 30 point scale) and a "category fluency" test (e.g., how many different animals the patient can name in one minute). In this small study, B vitamins appeared to slow cognitive and clinical decline in people with MCI, in particular in those individuals with elevated homocysteine. Further studies are warranted to determine whether these vitamins may slow or prevent the progression from MCI to AD.

In the area of AD treatment, a small research study showed increased clinical benefit of the FDA-approved drugs called cholinesterase-inhibitor medications when folic acid was used in combination (*International Journal of Geriatric Psychiatry*, 2008). For more information on treatment considerations for people already diagnosed with AD, see Chapters 22 through 26 in Section 4 of this book. As with all interventions, adding folic acid to a treatment plan needs to be discussed and approved by the treating physician.

A recent study published in the journal *Archives of Neurology* in 2012 by Galasko and colleagues found that the antioxidant combination of vitamin E, C, and alpha-lipoic acid (when taken in pill form) was found to have no effect on Alzheimer's patients (spinal fluid lab results improved slightly but memory function actually worsened slightly). In addition, another supplement called CoQ10 (coenzyme Q10) also had no effect. Past studies have shown benefits of eating a diet rich in antioxidants and certain vitamins, but this study did not show benefit of these specific antioxidants via pill/supplement form. More studies are needed to clarify these results in people already diagnosed with AD.

AN OVERVIEW OF SUPPLEMENTS FOR AD SUPPORTED BY RESEARCH

There are two types of supplements that have the most evidence in Alzheimer's treatment and prevention. The one with the most evidence is the class called omega-3 fatty acids, which is most commonly found in fish oil. The other is curcumin. Each of these will be discussed in more detail below. In addition, exciting new study findings suggest that cocoa powder has memory-promoting effects. We'll take a look at that as well before this chapter closes.

DEFINITION: **Dietary Supplements**

Dietary supplements, also referred to as nutraceuticals, are products that do not require a prescription from a physician, and are intended to supplement the diet and maintain good health and regular function. A supplement can contain any one or the combination of the following ingredients: vitamins, minerals, herbs or other botanicals, amino acids, dietary substances used to supplement the diet by increasing the total dietary intake (e.g., enzymes from tissues or organs), or a concentrate, metabolite, constituent, or extract.

Supplements are available from a variety of sources, including supermarkets, health food stores, drugstores, and on the Internet. For a listing of supplements and their evidence for AD treatment and prevention, visit www.therapy-formemory.org. When looking at the label of any supplement that makes a claim of an effect on structure or function of the body, expect to find the following: "This statement has not been evaluated by the FDA. This product is not intended to diagnose, treat, cure, or prevent any disease." For additional information on supplements, read about the term "dietary supplement" as defined by the Dietary Supplement Health and Education Act (DSHEA) of 1994, or visit www.Medical-NutritionFacts.com. Certain brands of supplements are of higher quality than others, but since the FDA does not specifically regulate their content, it is difficult for consumers to know the exact differences. In Dr. Isaacson's clinical practice, he tends to suggest brands that have the most optimal doses based on science and those with which his patients have had the most experience.

FISH OIL FOR AD TREATMENT AND PREVENTION

Fish oil has been studied in a variety of scientific trials, and there is evidence for its usefulness in Alzheimer's disease. There is some evidence that shows intake of specific types of fish oil may possibly delay the onset of the disease, as well as possibly improve or stabilize symptoms of AD.

One of the recommendations that we make as an adjunct to the dietary changes discussed earlier (e.g., low-carbohydrate, low saturated fat, high antioxidant) is to eat fish high in omega-3 fatty acids. More specifically, the types of omega-3 fatty acids we teach our patients about are docosahexaenoic acid (DHA), along with lesser amounts of eicosapentaenoic acid (EPA). There are several studies that show the potential benefit of these omega-3s (via diet and/or supplements) in AD. However, eating fish high in DHA and EPA, and taking DHA/EPA supplements, are not U.S. Food and Drug Administration (FDA) approved interventions for AD.

Based on evidence of effectiveness and safety, we have been recommending that our patients make specific dietary changes (including eating fish high in DHA and EPA) and consider complementing their diet with a nutritional supplement (in capsule or liquid form). After several years of making these recommendations, we are convinced that this approach is well tolerated, reasonably cost effective, and seems to be helpful in a number of patients (particularly those in the earliest stages of AD, as well as for possible prevention).

In terms of treatment, the most recent research has shown that it may be necessary for patients to take even higher amounts of DHA, such as 1,500–2,000 mg each day. This is based on a study published in *Archives of Neurology* in 2006 (DHA 1,720 mg and EPA 600 mg each day) that showed benefits, and another more recent trial that was performed by the Alzheimer's Disease Cooperative Study.

Currently, there is not enough high-quality research (i.e., prospective, randomized, double-blinded, placebo-controlled trials) to allow clinicians to say with 100 percent certainty which AD patients, if any, will surely respond to DHA. Although there is still much research to be done to determine what types work best, we suggest increasing dietary omega-3s from fish in combination with one of three specific types of supplements. In order to get a sufficient amount of DHA, Dr.

Isaacson tends to recommend a brand called Carlson Super DHA Gems, which have 500 mg of DHA per capsule. The benefit of this brand is based on the high amount of DHA per capsule balanced with a reasonable cost. Another brand is Life's DHA (made by Martek, and derived from algae—not fish). The benefit of this brand is that some of the most rigorous scientific studies used this exact brand of fish oil in their clinical trials. For both the Carlsons and Martek brands, many of Dr. Isaacson's patients have used and tolerated these well for many years. That being said, any brand with a high DHA content may also be substituted at the discretion of the treating physician.

More on DHA Fish Oil

The most recent study on using fish oil in the treatment of AD was published in the *Journal of the American Medical Association* in November 2010. This study used fish oil derived from algae (made by Martek) and found that 2,000 mg of DHA alone did not help patients when looked at as a group, but *did* help a subset of patients with a specific genetic makeup (APOE4 negative, see Chapter 15 for more details about genetics and Alzheimer's disease). Up to 45 percent of AD patients are APOE4 negative, and as such, even though most clinicians do not perform genetic testing, they may recommend the use of DHA supplements. Further studies in the future may help to clarify in which patients the different types of supplements (and vitamins) will work best.

Data published in November 2010 in *Alzheimer's and Dementia*, the journal of the Alzheimer's Association), showed that adults over the age of fifty-five with age-related cognitive decline demonstrated improvements in memory skills after taking 900 mg of algae-based DHA supplements each day (made by Martek). As an alternative to capsules, liquid fish oil may be used. One brand to consider is called Nutri Supreme (available online at www.nutri-supreme.com or by calling 1-888-68-NUTRI), which is also kosher. This brand is suggested as it is also relatively high in DHA, reasonably priced, and many of Dr. Isaacson's patients have used this for many years.

When visiting the supermarket, nutrition store, or neighborhood drugstore, there will usually be many types of fish oil available. As stated earlier, it is important to realize that all fish oils are not the same. The most common types will say "Fish Oil 1,000 mg" on the label. It is important to note that for possible prevention or delay of Alzheimer's disease, patients need to take the right type of fish oil (capsules or liquid) and in adequate amounts. It is advised to look at the label and see the breakdown of how much DHA and EPA are in each serving, and how many capsules are needed for each serving size. Oftentimes, individuals will need to take at least two or three servings each day, or more, in order to get a suitable amount of these two omega-3 fatty acids.

In general, fish oil supplements must have DHA and EPA in them (the more DHA the better). Try to get at least 250 mg of DHA in each capsule, and as mentioned earlier, aim for a total of at least 1,000–1,500 mg daily of DHA specifically. Fish oil should be started only under the supervision of a physician, and patients should try one capsule at first each day with a big meal and with water or juice. Then, if tolerated, increase to one capsule twice per day after a week or so. It is suggested to start low and increase slowly, until an adequate total dose of DHA/EPA is achieved.

While there is much research that needs to be done to replicate the findings mentioned above and clarify which types of fish oil work best, this evidence has led us to recommend fish oil supplements to patients at risk for AD. This is based on several studies. DHA supplementation, as was previously discussed above regarding AD treatment, fish oil may more optimally be used for prevention (or for delaying the onset of cognitive decline) in patients who are negative for the APOE4 gene. Further research is necessary to clarify this pharmacogenomic consideration.

DEFINITION: **Pharmacogenomics**

The study of how the same therapies may be more or less effective for different individuals due to differences in their genetic makeup.

Cost and Safety of Fish Oil Supplements

The cost of fish oil supplements depends on a variety of factors. The price most significantly depends on the brand or strength of the fish oil and the location purchased. There is often a price difference between pharmacies in the same town and on Internet websites. It is advisable to shop around and visit several pharmacies, health food stores, and websites, and discuss with other caregivers, a social worker, or staff at the treating physician's office.

It is imperative to pay close attention to the exact brand name, strength of each capsule, and serving size. The average cost of Carlson Super DHA Gems ranges from $30–$35 for 180 capsules, or $20–$25 per month (1,500 mg total DHA per day, 500 mg capsules), and the average cost of Life's DHA by Martek ranges from $22–$30 for 90 capsules, or $25 per month (900 mg total DHA per day, 300 mg capsules). As one example, the average cost for a 12-ounce bottle of the Nutri-Supreme "Omega-3 GOLD" liquid fish oil (also contains 1,000 IU of vitamin D3 per teaspoon) is $43, or roughly $35 per month via the manufacturer's website. If looking to purchase supplements, it may be a good idea to check websites such as ebay.com or amazon.com, where bulk orders may be less expensive. Purchasers must be careful to make sure the product is *exactly* what they are looking for.

As mentioned earlier, fish oil is generally safe but must be used under the supervision of a physician as there could be

OMEGA-3S FROM FOOD VERSUS SUPPLEMENTS

We always advocate for our patients to try to get as much of their brain-protecting nutrients from actual food, rather than a dietary supplement in pill or liquid form. The scientific evidence supports this concept. A recent study from 2012 by Tan and colleagues from UCLA showed that eating a diet rich in omega-3 fatty acids can protect against premature brain aging and memory loss. Researchers found that people with low omega-3s in their blood had less brain volume and scored lower on memory tests, compared with others with high omega-3s. This was published in the journal *Neurology* and was the first study to link blood levels of healthy fats to brain size and memory loss.

interactions with other medications the patient is taking. Fish oil may have an effect on bleeding and must be used with caution in people who are on anticoagulant (blood thinner) medications like Coumadin (must have blood work monitored by a physician on a regular basis). Overall, fish oil is generally safe and also may have a beneficial effect on cholesterol, so Dr. Isaacson does utilize this strategy frequently in his practice.

CURCUMIN (TURMERIC ROOT)

The other supplement that Dr. Isaacson often suggests to his patients is curcumin (aka turmeric root), which is the active ingredient in curry. There is no clear standardized dosing, and it is not currently known what dose or type is most beneficial. Ongoing scientific trials are studying this treatment, but since curcumin is generally safe and there is some data to suggest its usefulness, Dr. Isaacson recommends it in his clinical practice. Dr. Isaacson routinely suggests that his patients take each dose of curcumin with some amount of fat in a meal, as this may help with absorption. Taking curcumin at the same time as a fish oil supplement, which contains fatty acids, is one easy way of abiding by this recommendation.

Curcumin capsules can usually be purchased in a health food store, and the directions on the bottle should always be followed. Since the FDA does not regulate supplements, and all brands are different in terms of dosage/strength, it is unclear which are best. In terms of safety, it is essential to make sure to discuss taking this supplement with the treating physician as there may be some potential for interactions with prescribed medications. The cost of curcumin varies widely depending on vendor, dosage, and strength, on average $10–$15 per month. Aside from taking a curcumin supplement, buying the actual curcumin spice from a grocery store and adding it to meals as preferred may also be beneficial over time. It is currently unclear whether a concentrated capsule form or the spice added to food would be more effective.

COCOA POWDER

An exciting new study released in August 2012 showed that patients with MCI who had regular intake of the strong

DR. ISAACSON:

This therapy deserves consideration for people with both MCI and Alzheimer's disease, as well as anyone who is at risk. As soon as I heard about the results of the randomized, double-blind, placebo-controlled trial mentioned above, I immediately advised several of my patients to order the exact type of cocoa powder proven in this trial to work (visit www.TheADplan.com/blog/wordpress for a direct link to the product studied). While most dark chocolate contains flavonoids, which may help to protect the brain, there is also a high amount of saturated fat and sugar that may have negative effects. As such, for both treatment and prevention, I am only recommending this specific dark chocolate powder for my patients, starting at 1 packet per day for 1 week, increasing to 2 packets per day (since that was the intermediate dose studied in the trial), as tolerated and as approved by their primary care physician.

antioxidants found in chocolate (from dark cocoa powder) had improvement in memory function, as well as blood pressure and insulin resistance. In this study, patients received one of three different amounts of cocoa powder, or a placebo with no active antioxidants. The two groups that received the middle and highest amounts of cocoa powder had positive results, compared to the other two groups.

This study was the first dietary intervention study (highest-quality double-blind, placebo-controlled trial) to show regular consumption of cocoa flavonols can improve memory function, most likely due to an improvement in insulin sensitivity. While further study is necessary for both patients with Alzheimer's disease as well as for those at risk, these are exciting results. Visit www.TherapyForMemory.org/vitamin for more details on this study and for a direct link to the type cocoa powder found to be effective.

SUPPLEMENTS THAT MAY BE EFFECTIVE IN PREVENTING OR TREATING AD	
NAME	**RECOMMENDED DAILY AMOUNT**
DHA Fish Oil	Prevention: 900–1,200 mg (or more); Treatment: 1,500–2,000 mg
Curcumin	Dose unclear; take with fish oil or some fat in the meal to improve absorption
Cocoa Powder	500–750 mg of Cocoa Flavonols

CHAPTER 8

Combining Nutrition with Exercise and Behavioral Enrichment

Aside from diet, one area to which we devote considerable attention is social and physical activity for the prevention and treatment of Alzheimer's disease. Study findings have suggested that social and physical activity interventions, combined with dietary modifications, may be protective to the brain and delay the development of AD.

Several recent studies have shown the positive benefits of physical activity (from regular exercise to household chores) in possibly reducing the risk of Alzheimer's and mental decline, even in people older than age eighty. To learn more, check out the following articles, which include interviews with Dr. Isaacson:

WebMD.com: http://www.webmd.com/alzheimers/news/20120418/any-exercise-may-cut-alzheimers-risk-at-any-age

Time.com: http://healthland.time.com/2012/04/19/ can-household-chores-help-prevent-alzheimers.

In addition to exercise alone, significant research on a combination of lifestyle approaches has been shown to be beneficial for staving off memory problems. For example, diet and behavioral enrichment have been studied in a variety of animals. Interestingly, as dogs get older, they have increasing likelihood to develop the condition canine cognitive dysfunction syndrome—otherwise known as "doggie Alzheimer's." They develop memory problems similar to humans with cognitive decline (although we would not expect them to be losing their keys or misplacing their cell phones!).

One study conducted over three years by Dr. Carl Cotman and colleagues at the University of California at Irvine looked at whether nutrition and diet interventions could possibly reduce aging in the brain and protect cognition in dogs. The study investigators wanted to determine whether dietary antioxidants would reduce oxidative damage in the brain cells.

DEFINITION: **Antioxidants**

Vitamins, minerals, and other nutrients that protect and repair cells from damage caused by free radicals. (See Chapter 12 for more information.)

The antioxidant diet in Cotman's study contained several foods that we recommend later (e.g., spinach) as well as supplements. This was in an effort to help protect the part of the brain cell responsible for energy production (mitochondria), which is affected in AD.

This study showed that diet combined with exercise (three times per week) and increased socialization (dogs could exercise and play together) maintained thinking skills after three years. The combination also protected brain cells from aging. Increases in an important protein called brain-derived neurotrophic factor (BDNF) was also most evident in this group, and approached levels found in younger animals. BDNF, which is also found in humans, helps support survival of brain cells and encourages the growth of new brain cells and brain connections. These studies were published in the *Journal of Neuroscience* and *Neurobiology of Aging*, by Dr. Cotman and colleagues.

While this study was performed on dogs, there is still an important take-home message of this research: The combination of exercise and behavioral enrichment acts synergistically with diet to optimize brain health and cognitive performance. Integrating socialization elements into exercise may turn out to be a key factor, although this aspect needs further study.

Translating these findings to humans is necessary and will take several years, but why wait? We will cover several lifestyle changes that can be made (with the approval of and review by the treating physician) that may reduce the likelihood of developing AD or delay the onset of symptoms of cognitive decline.

A variety of research has studied social interactions including social ties and networking, and their effects on cognitive functioning. We are unsure of why or how more rigorous social relationships may protect memory. One thought is that hormonal factors may mediate stress and thus be protective. The interactions between social, psychological, and physical activities are important, as they work in combination to maintain cognition and possibly protect from later decline. From an intervention perspective, multimodal programs that are integrated into everyday life will likely yield the most benefit.

Social engagement not only may delay onset of memory loss/dementia, but may also increase the chance of living

DR. ISAACSON:
The best advice I can give regarding staying active was shared with me by my friend Hector Elizondo, a fellow Yankee fan and colleague who has dedicated himself tirelessly toward helping patients and caregivers with AD. His mother suffered from Alzheimer's, his father was her devoted caregiver, and I was fortunate to spend some time with him a few years ago helping to raise awareness of AD. He simply said, "Stay engaged in life!" These are the exact words I say virtually every day to those who are worried about developing AD.

longer. A variety of studies support that social interaction is an important factor for optimal aging. Aging can come with obstacles to social engagement (e.g., lack of physical activity, stigma of cognitive decline leading a person to withdraw from social activities with friends).

Considering this, researchers have recently begun to study whether online social networking (e.g., Facebook) can help delay memory loss or even promote cognitive functioning. A new research study by Deters, Mehl, and colleagues aimed to figure out if online social networking tools on Facebook like "Status Updates" and "Newsfeed" entries could be a helpful and/or meaningful form of social integration. The study was supported by the Evelyn F. McKnight Brain Research Foundation and the results were promising.

For more information on Social Engagement for AD, read the interview with Dr. Isaacson in the article "More Facebook Friends, More Gray Matter in Brain?"

http://www.doctorslounge.com/index.php/news/hd/23905

For anyone who has difficulty staying engaged socially or has trouble motivating a loved one to stay active, we suggest a number of helpful tips. First, get the help of a qualified healthcare professional. Some people may benefit from the assistance of a personal trainer, counselor, or life coach. Getting family members involved in a healthy Alzheimer's lifestyle and using each other for motivation is one of the best ways to achieve success—healthy family/group dinners, exercise sessions, and social activities will help to keep everyone engaged. Remember the saying, "Rome wasn't built in a day." Try to choose one or two aspects on which to focus, start slowly, and realize that efforts now will absolutely be worth the reward later. There is no better investment than in the health of oneself or in the ones you care about!

SECTION 2:

PUTTING INFORMATION INTO ACTION

CHAPTER 9

Carbohydrate Concepts

As mentioned earlier, in thinking about nutrition, it is helpful to picture the body as a furnace. To have a long and steady flame, high-quality firewood is needed. If someone puts paper in a furnace, it will burn in a flash and the flame will go out quickly. Kindling is a little better than paper, but it will also burn too fast. In other words, there is no substitute for high-quality firewood. The same is true of fuel for the body. In this chapter, we go into greater detail about high-quality (low-glycemic) carbohydrates versus low-quality (high-glycemic) carbohydrates and their effects on the brain.

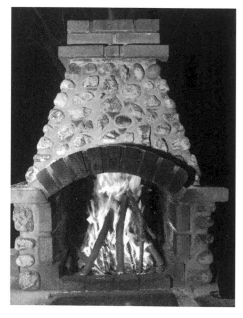

Several recent studies have shown that reducing carbohydrate intake can improve memory and more than likely also protect the brain. One study by Krikorian and colleagues (*Neurobiology of Aging*, 2010) aimed to determine the effects of dietary changes in patients with mild cognitive impairment (MCI). Patients with MCI were separated into two groups: one group was given a high-carbohydrate diet and the other a low-carbohydrate diet. After six weeks, patients who adhered to the low-carbohydrate diet demonstrated improved verbal memory performance, weight loss, decreased waist circumference, decreased blood sugar levels (high sugar levels may be harmful), and decreased fasting insulin (more on this later).

A similar study was performed in patients already diagnosed with Alzheimer's disease by Craft and colleagues (*Archives of Neurology*, 2011). These researchers compared two different types of dietary interventions on cognitive outcomes in AD patients: a Western-style diet (diet consisting of high saturated fat and high-glycemic index carbs) versus a Mediterranean-style diet (diet consisting of low saturated fat and low-glycemic index carbohydrates).

The results of this study were quite interesting. Those subjects who followed the Mediterranean-style diet did better in terms of memory function. It was suggested that the low-fat and low-carbohydrate diet improved memory in the study subjects, possibly due to positive effects on inflammation, oxidative stress, insulin, and other brain markers (beta-amyloid protein accumulation).

DEFINITION: **Oxidative Stress**

An imbalance in brain or other cells that can cause impairment in the body's ability to detoxify itself, whereby resulting in cellular damage

APPLYING THE CONCEPTS OF GLYCEMIC INDEX AND GLYCEMIC LOAD FOR A BRAIN-HEALTHY DIET

Although we touched upon the terms "glycemic index" and "glycemic load" in Section 1 of this book, let's take a closer look at the definitions of these key concepts.

"Glycemic index" is an actual number assigned to a particular food that represents the amount of insulin released after eating. This is also called insulin response. In other words, *glycemic index* refers to how quickly the specific food "spikes" or increases an individual's blood sugar (also called blood glucose) levels—basically, how quickly the food is "burnt up" in his or her furnace.

The glycemic index is also a marker of how quickly a specific food is processed through the body. High-glycemic index foods produce a rapid spike in blood glucose levels, which is typically followed by a "crash," or rapid decrease in blood glucose. In the United States, lunch is typically made up of high-glycemic index foods, and this crash is often felt around 2:00 p.m. Sound familiar? Not only may this crash leave a person feeling run down, but also consider the following:

1. High-glycemic index foods require no energy to digest (e.g., no calories are burned while digesting them).

2. We have only a certain amount of glucose that we can use toward providing us with energy at any one time (if the food is digested quickly, we rapidly reach the capacity of glucose we can use for energy and the rest is stored as fat).

Low-glycemic index foods, on the other hand, have a slower and more even rate of absorption during digestion, which means the foods are more gradually broken down. Low-glycemic index foods include fresh veggies, eggs, lean meat, whole grains, and some fresh fruits.

The term "glycemic load" takes the concept of glycemic index a step further by incorporating the relative amount of carbohydrate provided by a particular food. Thus, it is a measure of the glycemic index (quality) of the carbohydrate provided by the food *combined* with the actual amount of the carbohydrate. Many nutrition experts feel that this is a better measure than glycemic index because some foods may be high-glycemic index but provide very little carbohydrate in a typical serving and are, therefore, brain-healthy choices (e.g., raw carrots and watermelon).

The following are examples of glycemic index versus glycemic load: According to glycemic index, you should avoid carrots and eat sweet potatoes. Although carrots are high-glycemic index, they provide very little carbohydrate so the actual insulin response is relatively small (a good thing). On the other hand, sweet potatoes are relatively low-glycemic index but provide a large carbohydrate load, eliciting a large insulin response (a bad thing).

Thus, according to glycemic index, you should avoid certain fruits and vegetables, with which most nutrition experts would not agree. When considering the quality (glycemic index) *and* amount of carbohydrate (glycemic load), one finds that fresh fruits and vegetables are recommended.

CONCEPT 1: MINIMIZING HIGH-GLYCEMIC & CHOOSING LOW-GLYCEMIC FOODS

It's all about food choices! It's not always easy to make the right choice, but it is *always* doable. As an example, as part of a research study, Dr. Ochner ate at least one meal at McDonald's every day for two months and was able to eat low-glycemic index, low-glycemic load, low fat and low calorie for every meal purchased there. How? Choices! Specifically, he ate a grilled chicken snack wrap or grilled chicken sandwich (no mayo), and a side salad with fat-free dressing every day. The point is, anyone and everyone can make similar healthy choices; **they just need to make the decision to do it and stick with it**. Loopholes grow into gaping holes. Making a deal with oneself to always minimize glycemic index and glycemic load forces a person to find ways to follow a low-glycemic diet. After a while, that person will begin to feel like they are just eating healthy as opposed to "following a diet." We cannot stress the importance of this enough: when people feel like they are in "dietary jail," they will not be able to sustain the lifelong changes they want to make. **Everyone should take care not to have negative feelings toward their diet!**

Our patients often struggle with decreasing carbohydrates in their diets. However, it is important not to underestimate the importance of carbohydrate reduction over time. It is

86

human nature to respond better to immediate consequences of our actions, since this is how our brains are wired. Humans are able respond to delayed consequences (reward or punishments), but this is difficult for most people, especially when it comes to diet. If smoking caused a person's teeth to turn brown and lungs to shrivel up right away, chances are it would not be the leading cause of preventable death in the United States. If people became obese upon eating their first Big Mac, chances are obesity would not be the second cause of preventable death in the United States. If people became physically fit the first time they used the gym, there would likely be a lot fewer unused memberships at Bally's. If following a particular diet were easy or the effects seen immediately, everyone would have a "perfect" body, be as healthy as possible, and have maximal memory function. However, this is not the case. **With dietary changes, people will not see the effects right away.** It is important for dieters to be prepared for this and be willing to accept this fact.

We encourage reducing carbohydrate intake slowly but surely, and sustaining these changes over time to best preserve and protect memory. While scientific studies have shown that it may take patients already diagnosed with AD or those with MCI six weeks to have significant differences in brain and body function (as discussed earlier), it may be extremely difficult to objectively quantify improvements in the real world. The added bonus is that such dietary changes have been shown to protect the heart, and most who stick with it will feel better, have more energy, and will minimize the chance of developing obesity.

Particularly in the beginning, following a new diet requires time and effort. **If people look for ways to get**

around their diet, they will find them. When a person is fully committed to making the diet work, he or she will be successful and form a new relationship with food that will last forever. In addition, research indicates that a low glycemic diet may also improve health outcomes associated with many of the most common chronic conditions (e.g., diabetes, heart disease, high blood pressure).

From educating and motivating countless individuals over the years to change the way they think about and take in food, we have found the following to be true:

1. Those who follow the suggestions will derive health and wellness benefits that are in line with the effort they put in.

2. Those who are able to make changes that can be sustained (not changes that make them feel like they are being punished or limited) will have greater long-term success.

Remember, sustainability is key!

Why Is It so Hard to Reduce Carbohydrates, Especially Sugar?

Eating sugar triggers the reward-related areas of the brain, largely through release of a brain chemical (neurotransmitter) called dopamine. In fact, both sugar and cocaine trigger dopamine release from similar brain areas (Lee and colleagues, 2011, *Neuroscience*). We experience pleasurable and rewarding sensations from this stimulation and want to repeat these behaviors (eating more sugar and/or abusing cocaine) again and again.

The similarities between sugar and cocaine do not stop

there. In fact, the similarities are so many and striking, researchers are talking more and more about the possibility of "sugar addiction." For example, withdrawal symptoms commonly reported by substance abusers deprived of their drug of choice have been seen in mice allowed to binge on sugar solutions and then deprived of it, including teeth

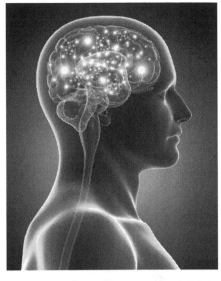

chattering and head shakes (Avena and colleagues, 2009, *Journal of Nutrition*). Similarly, people trying to cut back on high-fat and sugar-containing foods report unpleasant physical and psychological sensations, including sweating, headaches, and restlessness (Ifland and colleagues, 2009, *Medical Hypotheses*). Chronic overconsumption of sugar also resembles chronic substance abuse in its continued occurrence, despite medical and health consequences. Similar to chronic alcohol abusers who stand at higher risks for liver and cardiovascular disease, overconsumption of sugar significantly increases risk of insulin resistance, obesity, heart disease, and potentially AD.

CONCEPT 2: FOOD PREPARATION AS MEANS TO LOW-GLYCEMIC EATING

One of the best ways to learn and follow a low-glycemic diet is to cook as much of the food one eats as possible. Individuals learn by doing, because they will see what ingredients are in favorite foods and thus better understand what to watch out for. In addition, after becoming a preparer of food, one will become more mindful of what less optimal ingredients should be substituted or left out entirely of food prepared at restaurants. Cooking enables a person to follow the Alzheimer's Diet better because of the 100 percent control of what goes into meals. Self-preparation of food accomplishes the following:

1. Reduces worrying about how something is prepared (e.g., are those vegetables sautéed in oil, turning them from a healthy side dish into a dish that delivers as much fat and calories as a slice of birthday cake?).

2. Minimizes concern about whether particular essential ingredients are used or not (e.g., cooking spray instead of oil).

3. Limits confusion or indecision about what to order when dining out, since there is no embarrassment associated with placing complicated orders.

All of these obstacles are addressed in greater detail in the following section (concept 3). The take-home point here is that **at home, the food preparer is the sole master of dietary destiny**.

The Home Food Environment

Probably the most important element to low-glycemic food preparation at home is what is called the home food environment. A home food environment describes what foods and ingredients are available in the home, both good and bad. The reason people who eat out more often are more likely to be obese than those who eat most of their meals at home is that the general food environment in the United States and other developed nations is extremely poor. This is due to unhealthy, calorie-dense, fatty, high-glycemic foods being read-

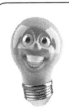

> **KEY CONCEPT:**
> Eliminate saturated fats and *bad* carbs (not *all* carbs!)

ily available (easy for restaurants to both get and store), cheap, and served quickly. Conversely, healthier (low-glycemic, low-fat, and low-calorie) options are typically harder to find and more expensive. This is one of the primary reasons that obesity rates spike whenever a particular locale becomes industrialized.

A good home food environment is one where healthy (low-glycemic, low-fat, and low-calorie) options are plentiful and unhealthy (high-glycemic, high-fat, and high-calorie) options are scarce. In essence, make your home food environment the opposite of the food environment outside!

> **KEY CONCEPT:**
> Make brain-healthy dietary changes that your taste buds won't notice!

Several dietary changes can be made with only minimal effort (e.g., selecting

ALTERNATIVE CHOICES

INSTEAD OF	USE
Oil	Cooking spray
Regular dairy products (i.e., mayonnaise, milk, cheese,	Fat-free (or at least reduced-fat) dairy products*, unsweetened almond or soy milk
Potato chips, pretzels, and other processed snack foods	Nuts, olives, cheese (low-fat or non-fat, goat or cottage), carrot sticks, hard-boiled eggs
Cold cereals	Yogurt parfait, steal-cut oatmeal, fiber-rich cereals
White pasta	Whole-wheat or brown-rice pasta, quinoa, spaghetti squash, zucchini slices
White rice	Brown or Basmati rice
Mashed potatoes	Mashed turnips, mashed cauliflower
French fries	Cucumbers, celery, green leafy vegetables, low-fat string cheese, carrot sticks
White bread or anything refined	Sprouted grain, stone ground, rye and pumpernickel bread*
Beer, grain alcohol	Red wine
White or milk chocolate	Dark chocolate, especially cocoa powder
Sugar	Stevia (natural sugar substitute)
Butter	Extra-virgin olive oil or cooking spray
Heavy cream	Fat-free half and half
Salad dressing	Olive oil, vinegar, lemon juice, salt and pepper
Cream cheese or butter on a bagel	Sugar-free jam or fat-free cream cheese on a bagel
Bacon	Canadian bacon, turkey bacon, or lean ham
Ricotta cheese	Low-fat or non-fat cottage cheese

INSTEAD OF	USE
Mayonnaise on a sandwich	Mustard or avocado
Croutons	Walnuts
Iceberg lettuce	Romaine lettuce
Sour cream	Yogurt (unsweetened)
Juice	Half juice and half water
Soda	Diet soda, water
Ice cream	Sorbet, sugar-free low-calorie frozen yogurt
Ground beef	Lean ground turkey
Hamburger on bun	Veggie burger on lettuce wrap
High fructose corn syrup	Maple syrup, agave nectar
Flour	Ground nuts
Macaroni and cheese	Whole-wheat pasta with mixed vegetables and parmesan cheese

* Whole wheat bread is mediocre, and enriched is not all that rich. See the Food Terminology guide in Appendix B for more details.

sugar-free or reduced-fat ingredients) while not detracting from the pleasure of the foods. There have been scientific studies proving that people cannot tell the difference between regular meals and meals cooked with reduced-fat ingredients. For example, Gruen and colleagues presented findings at the American Chemical Society meeting that research subjects liked low-fat chocolate ice cream as much as full-fat ice cream (1999). This is certainly not to say that all or even the majority of sugar-free or fat-free products taste like their regular counterparts. However, it is extremely difficult to discern differences between *meals* cooked with fat-free, low-fat, and/or sugar-free *ingredients* versus regular meals.

People following the Alzheimer's Diet do not have to give up their favorite high-glycemic foods entirely. Instead, we recommend eating them in moderation and balancing them with proteins, unsaturated fats, and low-glycemic carbohydrates.

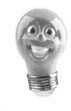

KEY CONCEPT: Everyone should eat what they enjoy eating!

Of course it is not okay to stuff oneself with pizza and cheeseburgers every day. That is not what we are saying. When we say that people should eat what they enjoy eating, we mean that they should find a way to prepare their favorite foods so they are lower in glycemic index and load (as well as saturated fat, which will be covered in the next chapter). Lowering the glycemic index and load of one's favorite food items is not only doable, but it can also be an exciting challenge from which to later benefit. Again, once this becomes habit, individuals turn into brain-healthy food gurus for the rest of their lives.

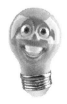

KEY CONCEPT: There are always ways to make a meal "brain healthier." These subtle changes in diet can help protect the brain over time.

DR. OCHNER:

*Personally, I still have the taste buds of a five-year-old. I frequently eat foods like pizza, burgers, and ice cream. No matter what the health ramifications, I would not be able to maintain a diet that did not contain these foods. I just love food too much, and I'm pretty sure there are other people who feel the same way. Here's the secret: eat the foods you enjoy eating, just make them healthy. There is no rule or law saying that pizza, burgers, or even hot fudge sundaes necessarily have to be high in glycemic load, saturated fat, and calories. Most of your favorite foods can be **prepared** so they are brain-healthy. Following are a few of my favorite examples.*

PIZZA PIZAZZ—A BRAIN HEALTHIER VERSION OF PEPPERONI PIZZA

1 Flatbread from Trader Joe's

12 slices turkey pepperoni

$1/2$ cup tomato sauce (no sugar added)

$1/2$ cup fat free mozzarella cheese

$1/8$ cup mix of oregano, black pepper, crushed red pepper, and parsley

	REGULAR PEPPERONI PIZZA	FLATBREAD PEPPERONI PIZZA
Serving size	2 slices	1 flatbread pizza
Calories	814	390
Total fat	36 g	4 g
Saturated fat	16 g	1 g
Carbohydrates	86 g	48 g
Sugar	8 g	6 g

Glycemic index	51	30
Glycemic load	43	14

BOCA IS BETTER—BRAIN-HEALTHY BIG MAC SUBSTITUTE

2 slices whole-grain toast or (preferably) 1 whole-grain bun

1 Boca burger patty (note: contains large amounts of gluten)

$1/4$ cup shredded lettuce

1 slice fat-free American cheese

2 tbsp adapted special sauce ($1/8$ recipe below)

$1/2$ cup fat-free mayonnaise

3 tablespoons fat-free French salad dressing

2 tablespoons sweet pickle relish (no sugar added)

1 teaspoon sugar substitute (e.g., stevia)

1 teaspoon dried, minced onion

1 teaspoon white vinegar

1 teaspoon ketchup

	McDonald's Big Mac	Boca Alternative
Serving size	1 burger	1 burger
Calories	550	295
Total fat	29 g	2 g
Saturated fat	10 g	0 g
Carbohydrates	46 g	34 g
Sugar	9 g	6 g
Glycemic index	51	38
Glycemic load	23	13

I SCREAM, YOU SCREAM, WE ALL SCREAM FOR A BRAIN-HEALTHY HOT FUDGE ICE CREAM SUNDAE

1 cup sugar-free ice cream

4 tablespoons calorie-free fudge topping (Not only does this exist, but it actually tastes good. Check specialty food stores.)

2 tablespoons fat-free whipped cream

	REGULAR HOT FUDGE SUNDAE	BRAIN-HEALTHY HOT FUDGE SUNDAE
Serving size	1 sundae	1 sundae
Calories	480	228
Total fat	26 g	4 g
Saturated fat	18 g	0 g
Carbohydrates	55 g	2 g
Sugar	42 g	1 g
Glycemic index	49	2
Glycemic load	27	1

DR. OCHNER:

Could I tell the difference between the regular and brain-healthy versions if I were blindfolded? Probably. But the difference is not nearly as alarming as one would think. And here is the most interesting part; I actually have grown to prefer the adapted brain-healthy versions. Why? Because most of these things I eat are actually good for me, so I am getting high-quality protein and nutrients without any of the saturated fat and most of the simple carbs. Any minimal amount that may be given up in taste is more than gained back by the fact that I get to eat my favorite kinds of foods all the time, completely guilt-free. In fact, better than guilt-free, I enjoy them more because I know I am eating something good for my body and brain!

CONCEPT 3: OVERCOMING CHALLENGES IN LOW-GLYCEMIC EATING

As mentioned, revamping dietary habits and sticking to a healthy plan is not easy; otherwise everyone would do it. A lot of this comes down to a decision to stick with it. Ask anyone who has quit smoking! Approaching dietary changes without a firm commitment from the outset will tend to result in a short "attempt" at making dietary changes, followed by a reversion back to old habits. Those who approach dieting this way will wind up frustrated and blame the diet for their failure. *The Alzheimer's Diet* represents the most current science in relation to nutrition, memory loss, and neurodegenerative (brain) disease. However, success will be measured more so by how well individuals are first educated about healthy food choices, and then how well they apply this new-found information in their daily lives. There is no aspect to a diet, no tip, no trick, no technique, more important than the decision to **stick to it.**

We cannot stress this enough. That being said, we know it is not always easy, and there will be challenges along the way. Below are some common challenges to adhering to this diet and some suggestions on how to deal with them. Just remember that as long as people are committed to making the change, they will find that arriving at solutions is not as difficult as they imagined. Finding individually tailored solutions is always best.

"I have kids and I have to have junk food for them."

This is a common obstacle to creating the ideal home food environment. Remember, we are much more likely to eat things we know we should not when they are readily available. One idea is to ration them. Places cookies and other brain-unhealthy snacks in separate plastic bags and put the kids' (or spouse's) name on them. It will be much harder to *steal* Bobby's or Jessica's favorite snack than it would be to take a cookie from the package.

"I cook for my husband who doesn't want to follow a low-glycemic plan."

Ideally, every individual in the household will be on board with brain-healthy eating. Done correctly, they should not even notice a difference in most prepared foods! We want our loved ones to be in the best overall health possible, in order for them to function at their best and feel healthy.

If it is not possible to slip low-glycemic meals by family

> **DR. OCHNER:**
> I hated the fact that I was the only kid in grade school whose lunch sandwiches were made with whole-wheat bread instead of the squishy Wonder bread that could be rolled up into little balls. Eventually, I caught on and realized that Mom knew best.

members, an important compromise is to limit the tempting high-glycemic foods kept in the house. If family members make specific requests for these items, there may be times where it could be helpful to prepare separate meals. Individuals also may choose to use a meal replacement (most people replace breakfast, but which meal is replaced is entirely up to the individual).

"I don't have time to cook" or "I eat most of my meals on the go."

Meal replacements are perfect for busy individuals who frequently eat on the go. For the meals that are not replaced, the person will need to choose wisely. This will require attention and effort in the beginning. However, as long as individuals stick to the diet, they will come to easily recognize the low-glycemic options at favorite restaurants and likely find new restaurants that present more low-glycemic options. As they say, "Necessity is the mother of all invention." As long as straying from a brain-healthy diet is not an option, each person will figure out what and where to eat fairly quickly. See tips in Chapter 20 for brain-healthy eating while outside of the home. Also, check online for the nutrition facts for meals at frequented chain restaurants; they are almost always available. This is where the investment in some initial investigatory work comes into play. There are too many potential options to cover here, but we hope that readers will be invested and curious enough to seek this information out.

It is also important to note that preparing meals at home (even bagged lunches) does not take nearly the amount of time or effort that most people think. Even at dinner, research from Beck and colleagues at UCLA has shown that with the right ingredients in the pantry and fridge, preparing a meal takes only about *ten minutes* more than making a trip to buy fast food, costs less, and is much healthier (*British Food Journal*, 2007).

"A low-glycemic diet is too expensive."

Incorporating meal replacements into the diet can help keep costs down. Also, while there aren't as many low-glycemic bulk products available as there are high-glycemic products, healthier choices are available if you know how to look for them. This is an area where the training and effort put forth in the 9-Week Diet Plan will come into play (see Chapter 18 for more information on this). Those following a brain-healthy diet will begin to know what to look for and will be able to choose brain-healthy foods at almost any store or restaurant while still keeping cost in mind.

We cannot tell people exactly what to buy since grocery purchases depend on individual tastes, but we can suggest some stores that we know have inexpensive solutions. These stores include Trader Joe's and warehouse stores such as Costco, Sam's Club, and BJ's. Shopping at such stores is a good opportunity to stock up on low-glycemic foods that may otherwise be cost prohibitive. In addition, make regular trips to the supermarket to scan for sales on brain-healthy items and stock up when there is a bargain. Again, with a little patience and effort in the beginning, people will find that there is no reason a brain-healthy diet needs to be any more expensive than a regular diet.

DR. OCHNER:

In college, my challenge was eating very high protein and very low fat at the same time with a $100/month food and entertainment budget. From this experience, I can tell you that it is definitely doable.

"I don't want to give up my favorite foods!"

We say, "Don't!" It is best to find ways to turn favorite foods into brain-healthier options. For those few foods that cannot be made more brain-healthy, enjoy them in moderation. Also, be patient with the diet. As new habits develop, taste preferences will follow accordingly.

CONCEPT 4: GLYCEMIC GUIDE: GOOD VERSUS BAD CARBOHYDRATES

The low-carb diet craze of the late nineties has started to dwindle. This is because, as with almost every "fad diet," science and the general public have discovered that it is not a magic cure for anything. Further, it was a radical diet that was difficult to maintain. Like nearly all weight-loss diets, the low-carb diet was effective in the short term, but many people could not stick to it, and the weight (and negative medical consequences that come with excess weight) soon returned.

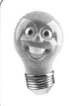

KEY CONCEPT: Carbohydrates are not necessarily bad!

Thus, we want to be very clear that we are not promoting a "fad" or crash diet to whip one's memory into shape for the summertime or any other season. What we propose here is to

DR. OCHNER:

*As a kid, there was nothing I enjoyed more than a huge pile of chicken nuggets and fries. We would go to McDonald's, get a twenty-piece nugget meal and "biggie" fry, and dump them all together on our trays . . . right next to a **huge** pile of ketchup. Fast forward twenty years, and the thought of the hydrogenated corn oil, grease, high fructose corn syrup, and saturated fat that these food items ooze makes me ill to even think about. The same will happen over time for anyone on the Alzheimer's Diet. This is a good thing.*

make key dietary changes that can be sustained for the rest of one's life. We make a lot of specific suggestions and not everyone will want (or be able to) incorporate all of them. Don't worry! Find the ones that work best for you and incorporate them into daily living. Instead of thinking about it as "going on the Alzheimer's Diet," focus on the memory-improving lifestyle changes that will be enjoyed for years to come.

In general, good carbohydrates are complex carbohydrates. These are found in foods like whole grains, fruits, vegetables, nuts, seeds, legumes, and dairy products (just watch out for high fat content in dairy products). Note that many of these foods also contain large amounts of fiber and protein, which is also good. Conversely, bad carbohydrates are simple carbohydrates, such as sugar. Simple carbohydrates are found in foods like white bread, white rice, most desserts, cookies, candy and sugared beverages (do not forget about beverages!). Although we encourage the consumption of some good carbohydrates, it is important to note that overall carbohydrate intake (good and bad) is very important for a brain-healthy diet. In the 9-Week Diet Plan (Chapter 18), we lay out specific guidelines for total carbohydrate intake, regardless of whether they are good or bad carbohydrates. That said, the glycemic load provides a good guide for overall carbohydrate intake as well as how much each food will cause blood sugar to spike.

There are a number of available websites that list the glycemic load (and index) of almost every kind of food. The most comprehensive website seems to be: http://www.men-dosa.com/gilists.htm. This list can be useful to check the glycemic load of specific kinds of foods and to search for low-glycemic options and replacement ingredients. However, the relative comprehensive nature of this list means that it may be difficult for the beginning low-glycemic eater to tell which general types of foods they should eat more or less of and which foods make the "best" and "worst" lists. Once familiar with the concepts of glycemic load (and saturated fat, covered in the next chapter), less time will be spent looking things up. However, in the beginning, some effort will be required to become familiar with the essentials. In order to assist with this, we provide a quick-start guide below.

TOP 10 GREAT MEMORY FOODS:

1. Fish high in the Omega-3 fatty acid DHA (wild salmon, albacore, herring, sardines)

2. Berries (especially blueberries and strawberries)

3. Seeds/nuts (flaxseeds, walnuts, pecans)

4. Green, leafy vegetables

5. Cocoa powder

6. Legumes (small red beans, pinto beans, black beans)

7. Grape juice (no sugar added)

8. Curry (or curry powder, also called turmeric root)

9. Black or green tea

10. Dark-skinned fruits

TOP 10 POOR MEMORY FOODS:

1. White bread

2. Candy

3. Sugary beverages, such as soda and "whateverochino" coffee drinks from chain coffee shops (these drinks can often be prepared with less sugar and fat if requested)

4. Cakes and muffins

5. Most fried foods

6. Foods sautéed in high-fat, high-caloric vegetable or corn oil (extra-virgin olive oil, which contains more "heart-healthy" fat, isn't usually the oil of choice at most restaurants).

7. Most dried foods (e.g., potato chips, corn chips, crackers, and dried fruits with added sugar)

8. Bacon

9. Hot dogs

10. Buttered popcorn

CHAPTER 10

Fat Concepts

As you learned in the previous chapter, not all carbohydrates are created equal. The same is true for fats. Some fats are actually considered "good" fats primarily because they help raise "good" (HDL) cholesterol (among their other effects on the body). Although we do suggest increased intake of these good fats, we always stress moderation. As mentioned earlier, replacing dietary fat with refined carbohydrates had been a common dietary practice in the past. However, we now know that this trade off is not optimal and can actually be worse for 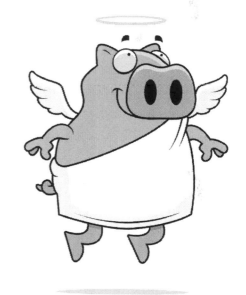 our bodies and brains. Shopping for good fats and keeping the diet low in fat overall can be a challenge, so in this chapter, we'll not only cover the basics about fat, we'll also discuss how to overcome the challenges to maintaining a brain-healthy low-fat diet.

CONCEPT 1: GOOD VERSUS BAD FAT

One of the primary goals of this chapter is to educate readers on the concepts behind "good" vs. "bad" fats. Briefly, unsaturated fats (monounsaturated and polyunsaturated) are considered good fats, while saturated fats and trans fats are considered bad fats. Intake of monounsaturated fats (e.g., extra virgin olive oil, peanuts, avocados) and polyunsaturated fats (e.g., nuts and seeds) in moderation is advisable. However, avoiding trans fats and reducing saturated fats are essential to maintaining a brain-healthy diet.

DEFINITION: Fat

Fat is the most calorically dense of the macronutrients. Fat contains 9 calories per gram (versus protein and carbohydrate, which contain only 4 calories per gram). Some fat is essential to proper functioning, but as with carbohydrates, all fats are not created equal.

DEFINITION: Trans Fat

Trans fats are linked to obesity, heart disease, accelerated aging, and cancer. They are difficult for the body to break down. Be aware that foods that advertise having "no trans fat" may still be high in saturated (and/ or unsaturated) fat and calories. In addition, FDA regulations allow food processors to claim "zero trans fats" on the label even if the food actually contains 0.49 grams (per serving). If individuals look at the ingredients, they will likely see partially hydrogenated oil, which is the primary source of trans fat.

DEFINITION: Saturated Fat

High intake of saturated fat is linked to heart disease, obesity, and some cancers. It can also raise LDL cholesterol (the "bad" cholesterol). There are a number of saturated fats, some safer than others. In general, however, it is a good idea to limit saturated fats.

DEFINITION: Polyunsaturated Fat

Polyunsaturated fat contains a balance of omega-3 and omega-6 fatty acids.

DEFINITION: Monounsaturated Fat

Sometimes called the "heart-healthy fat," monounsaturated fat can actually reduce the "bad" cholesterol (LDL).

DEFINITION: Extra-Virgin Olive Oil

Extra-virgin olive oil is produced from pressing the olives without the addition of solvents. Must have low free-acidity (less than 0.8 percent), which indicates higher quality. Still high in saturated fat and calories (so use small amounts) but shown to raise HDL ("good") cholesterol.

The "goodness" of a fat is heavily linked to its effect on cholesterol. Cholesterol is essential for building and maintaining membranes in the body. The body also needs cholesterol to make several important compounds, such as vitamin D, estrogen, and testosterone. Too much cholesterol is generally considered a bad thing, but **what is really important is actually an individual's ratio of good to bad cholesterol (HDL : LDL).** Low-density lipoproteins (LDL) transport cholesterol from the liver to the rest of the body. Excessive LDL causes plaque to build up on the walls of arteries throughout the body, which can limit blood flow and potentially break apart, causing heart attack or stroke. Conversely, high-density lipoproteins (HDL) actually collect cholesterol from artery walls and transport it back to the liver for disposal. **Bad fats (all trans fats and many saturated fats) generally raise LDL, while good fats (monounsaturated and polyunsaturated fats) generally lower LDL and raise HDL.**

FOODS HIGH IN BAD (SATURATED) FAT:

- Most fast foods

- Hydrogenated oil (palm, coconut; see Chapter 17 for more information on different types of coconut oil)

- Dried coconut

- Butter

- Animal fats (shortening, lard)

- Milk and white chocolate; dark chocolate (although it is rich in antioxidants)

- Cheese

FOODS HIGH IN GOOD (UNSATURATED) FAT:

- Certain oils when used in moderation (extra-virgin olive oil, peanut, hazelnut, canola, sesame, safflower, sunflower, soybean, corn)

- Avocados

- Olives

- Certain nuts (almonds, hazelnuts, walnuts, pecans, pistachios, cashews, macadamia)

- Peanut butter (although also high in saturated fat)

- Certain seeds (pumpkin, sesame, sunflower)

- Certain fish (wild salmon, sardines, tuna, mackerel, lake trout)

CONCEPT 2:
LOW- AND NON- FAT ITEMS—CHOOSE WISELY

Some low- and non-fat options *can* be great replacements for foods that would otherwise be harmful to one's body and memory. However, **caution must be taken when choosing reduced-fat options**. With relatively few exceptions, food manufacturers are watching out for their bottom line rather than the health of their customers. Many reduced-fat versions of packaged foods are simply smaller portions (so they contain less fat than full por-

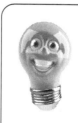

KEY CONCEPT: "Low fat" and "non fat" do not necessarily mean healthy!

tions). More commonly, and potentially more memory damaging, are the large proportion of low- and non-fat products that replace fat with excessive amounts of sugar and salt. **It is imperative to read the nutrition labels of low- and non-fat products to make sure that the carbohydrate content is acceptable, according to the targets outlined in the 9-Week Diet Plan.**

CONCEPT 3:
OVERCOMING CHALLENGES IN LOW-FAT EATING

Although some people will face challenges in low-fat eating, such as those described below, transitioning to a low-fat diet also provides the opportunity to make large improvements in the brain health of one's diet without sacrificing a lot of taste. Of course, not all low-fat products taste as good as their full fat counterparts; however, many of them do. We suggest experimenting with different low- and non-fat food items to see which ones taste the best. As mentioned earlier, just be sure to verify that they do not contain excessive amounts of sugar (and salt).

Knowing Where the Fat Is Challenge

Most people are ingesting far more fat, particularly saturated fat (and calories), than they realize. The worst part about this is that most people are not even enjoying a lot of the fat that they eat. They could be hurting their bodies and mind without even realizing it, and with little enjoyment. Particularly when beginning the Alzheimer's Diet, it is vital that people learn where the bad fats are hidden and how to eat around them. This is part of the reason we stress reading nutrition labels and creating brain-healthy versions of the person's favorite foods during the 9-Week Diet Plan. As individuals become familiar with the nutritional content of foods and ingredients in their favorite meals, they will begin to recognize hidden fat and learn how they can find or create the same foods without the bad fat.

Bad Habits/Mindless Eating Challenge

Bad habits can present a real roadblock when switching to a healthier diet. For example, many people practice "mindless eating." This means that they are not paying attention to (or really enjoying) their food when they are eating. For example, someone sits down in front of the TV or at computer, and the next thing they know, they have eaten a plate of food! Hopefully that food was low in saturated fat and glycemic load, but chances are it was not. When following the Alzheimer's Diet, it is important to pay a lot of attention not only to the food on the plate but also to the process of eating. This will require some conscious effort at first, but it does come with an added benefit; when people pay closer attention to something pleasurable (like eating), they actually enjoy it more! This means that **people following the Alzheimer's Diet should not only maintain the enjoyment they get from eating, but actually enjoy their diet more!**

The "Dietary Jail" Challenge

As mentioned previously, it is vital that a diet plan does not make a person feel like they are in dietary jail. We are intentionally repeating this concept because *it is essential to making lasting changes* in diet and brain health. In the 9-Week Diet Plan detailed in Chapter 18, we ask individuals to experiment with different brain-healthy food options, which include low saturated fat foods. Anyone who makes a commitment to finding good-tasting low saturated fat options is usually able to do so relatively quickly, while anyone who is resistant to this dietary change often feels that it is impossible and gives up after a couple of half-hearted attempts. People who put the initial effort into finding healthy options are more likely to maintain these improvements in their diet because they still enjoy eating. Eating should always be a pleasurable (and healthy) experience!

Remember, in terms of brain-healthy dietary changes, more is better, but a little is much better than nothing. Even if a person decided to follow only one or two recommendations in *The Alzheimer's Diet*, that person would still be making positive changes in terms of brain health. Substituting just one item high in saturated fat with a healthier counterpart could improve brain health over time. Of course, we hope that everyone who reads this book makes *many* small changes and discovers ways to make their diet more brain-healthy without reducing their overall enjoyment of food!

The "All-or-Nothing Thinking" Challenge

Chances are that eating is something we will all do every day for the rest of our lives. And, like most other things in life, there are ups and downs, good days and bad days. We want to discourage the common notion that a diet is "blown" if someone has a day—or even couple of days—of unhealthy (e.g., high saturated fat) eating. It is vital that individuals do not completely abandon a diet just because of one off day. That is the trap of all-or-nothing thinking.

Think about the stock market. Nothing moves in a perfectly straight line from A to B. **What is important is the change that takes place over time.** There will be days where one's diet is more brain-healthy (stock goes up) and days where one's diet is less brain-healthy (stock goes down). Even if some days bring the "stock value" of one's diet down, resuming a brain-healthy diet the next day will bring the value back up. Look at the Alzheimer's Diet this way and not as a diet that can be "gone off" or "blown." This is a program to help people figure out what brain-healthy changes work for them *most of the time*—not necessarily all of the time—for the rest of their lives.

CHAPTER 11

Protein Concepts

The human brain is composed of various parts that are responsible for different elements of life. For example, certain areas serve as "homeostatic" centers to keep us alive (e.g., regulating body temperature, respiration, and heart rate). Other areas are responsible for strength, balance, vision, coordination, and thought, for example. With all of the different areas that need to support each other, it is not unexpected that the body and brain require a variety of dietary components to function properly. When it comes to the "thinking" part of the brain, a balanced diet consisting of an optimal combination of carbohydrate, fat, and protein can help

KEY CONCEPT:
Do not underestimate the importance of protein for the brain.

keep our memory finely tuned. Of course this is addition to all of the other positive effects of a balanced diet on overall our health. In this chapter we discuss different forms of protein, what constitutes "high-quality" protein, common foods to maximize lean high-quality protein, and challenges to eating high-quality lean protein.

CONCEPT 1: DIFFERENT FORMS OF PROTEIN

Protein is protein, right? Wrong. There are several different forms of protein, and not all protein is created equal. (Sound familiar?) Similarly, not all protein is used by our bodies in the same way, as discussed in each of the following sections.

Animal versus Plant Protein

For those not as interested in the science behind it, the most important thing to remember is that animal protein (protein from fish, lean meat, etc.) is generally more easily utilized by the body relative to plant protein (protein from beans, vegetables, etc.). We mention a couple of exceptions below, but this is generally true. This has to do with the different amino acid profiles of each form of protein. Amino acids are the "building blocks" of protein in the human body. They are made up of carbon, hydrogen, oxygen, and nitrogen. All the major macronutrients (protein, fat, and carbohydrate) contain carbon, hydrogen, and oxygen. However, protein also contains nitrogen, which is necessary for the construction of amino acids. The different amino acid profiles of different forms of protein determine the rates at which the amino acids can be utilized by the body.

Animal proteins have structures more similar to natural human proteins than do plant proteins and are, therefore, easier for our bodies to put to work. The focus, however, should be on eating as much "high-quality" protein as possible, whether it comes from animals or plants (though more commonly found in animal protein). High-quality protein is discussed below.

Note: There is some research suggesting there may be a

connection between animal protein and cancer. The jury is still out on this, but some epidemiological studies (which take data from large groups of people and see if different conditions may be statistically related) support this finding. For example, self-reported frequency of red meat consumption and incidence of colorectal cancer suggests that individuals who consume the most animal protein may be at higher risk for certain types of cancer. That being said, most physicians do not feel that the risk is high enough to supersede the benefits of animal protein. However, each individual must make this decision for him- or herself and should discuss their dietary patterns with their treating physician (especially if there is a family history or individual past history of cancer).

High-Quality Protein

In short, protein from food is not the same as protein produced by our bodies. Protein produced by our bodies is necessary to support a variety of biological functions, including memory function. High-quality protein gives the body everything it needs to produce this "internal" protein. So where does one find high-quality protein? Lean meat, fish, egg whites, and low-fat or non-fat milk are some common examples. Despite the fact that animal protein is generally better than plant protein, soybeans, quinoa, and spinach are also considered high-quality protein.

The science behind this: The human body needs twenty "common" amino acids to produce the protein it needs to support normal body reactions and to build and repair cells and tissues. However, our body can only produce eleven of the twenty common amino acids on its own. Thus, we need the amino acids in protein from food in order for our bodies to produce the protein it needs. The nine common amino acids our body cannot produce by itself are considered "essential amino acids." Therefore, protein sources that are rich in those nine essential amino acids are considered high-quality protein.

Whey versus Soy versus Casein versus Egg Protein

As we have discussed, there are several different forms of protein. Each has a different biological value, net utilization value, efficiency ratio, and so on. We will talk a little about these things in more detail, but for those who just want the take-home message: **whey, soy, and egg-white protein are arguably the best forms of protein. Of these, most experts recommend whey protein.**

Whey protein is actually a collection of proteins that are isolated from whey, which is a byproduct of cheese manufactured from cow's milk (along with casein). It is the most common form of protein sold in protein supplements for good reason (discussed below) and is the general recommendation of most experts for individuals seeking additional manufactured protein in their diet.

As one might expect, soy comes from soybeans. There is much conjecture about the health benefits of soy protein and how it stacks up against other forms, particularly whey protein. Some studies suggest that soy protein is protective against some forms of cancer, while other studies suggest that high soy protein intake may be related to higher incidence of other forms of cancer. Similarly to the research on the potential connection between red meat and cancer, the data is mixed and unclear, and such dietary changes should be discussed with and approved by the treating physician.

Another form of protein called casein is an additional byproduct of cheese, and is manufactured from cow's milk. It tends to contain higher levels of lactose, which is a milk sugar, and causes digestive difficulties in a fair number of people. It is similar to cottage cheese but with a higher amount of lactose. It is relatively rare to find casein protein supplements, because whey and soy are almost universally considered superior.

As one would guess, egg protein is derived from eggs. Naturally occurring egg protein is derived from both the white and yolk of the egg. Be aware, however, that egg yolks are relatively high in saturated fat and cholesterol, while the whites are high in protein but have almost no fat or cholesterol. As such, there is a fair amount of popularity of egg-white products, especially since egg protein is a high-quality protein.

Of these protein sources, whey and egg protein have the highest biological value, which indicates the digestibility and bioavailability of the protein. Whey protein has the highest net protein utilization, which indicates the amount of amino acids that can be converted to protein inside the body. Whey protein also has the highest protein efficiency ratio, which the FDA uses to derive the recommended daily allowance (RDA). For these reasons, most people who utilize protein supplements will choose whey protein.

Note: Whey, soy, and egg proteins are all rich in the amino acids critical for muscle building and maintenance. This may be important for people who are also attempting to lose weight, as some amount of muscle loss is a nec-essary consequence of weight loss. Studies show that

119

reduced-calorie diets rich in the amino acids derived from these protein sources help preserve muscle and lead to a higher ratio of fat to muscle loss.

For individuals to max-imize the brain-healthy aspects of their diet, they must make a concerted effort to find *lean* high-quality protein. Several of these are suggested below.

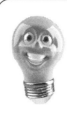

KEY CONCEPT: Protein and fat tend to be found together, so choose protein wisely.

CONCEPT 2: COMMON FOODS TO MAXIMIZE HIGH-QUALITY LEAN PROTEIN

The foods below are not only outstanding sources of high-quality protein, but they are also lean. This means that they provide very little, if any, saturated fat and relatively little total fat. These high protein foods also provide few carbohy-drates. Therefore, we recommend that the largest portion of a meal come from these components. For example, a brain-healthy dinner plate may be 60 percent lean protein (e.g., large piece of fish) and 40 percent green leafy vegetables.

Chicken

We do not mean chicken wings, chicken nuggets, or deep-fried chicken. Opt instead for white meat over dark meat, and organic if possible. Overall, almost any non-fried serving of chicken will provide an outstanding protein to calorie ratio (meaning it will deliver an outstanding "bang for your buck" in terms of how much one has to eat to get an adequate portion of protein). An important note about chicken skin—yes, the skin is that bad. Do not eat it whenever possible. And, yes, dark meat is higher in fat than white meat. In fact, dark meat has approximately twice the total fat and (worse) saturated fat as compared to white meat.

Turkey

Overall, turkey is similar to chicken. When purchasing turkey, be careful to avoid the addition of high and potentially unhealthy amounts of sodium. Remember to check the nutrition labels for serving size and types, as well as the ingredients of turkey products, to ensure quality.

Fish

Avoid fried fish or fish dishes that are sautéed in oil. If one has the financial means to be more selective, we suggest they opt for organic and/or wild-caught varieties. Particular types of fish, such as wild salmon, lake trout, herring, sardines, and mackerel are rich in high-quality protein, as well as brain-healthy omega-3 fatty acids (DHA).

We suggest choosing wild over farm-raised salmon for a variety of reasons, but mainly due to the higher content of DHA. However, in addition to the DHA benefit, a study by Hites and colleagues found that farm-raised salmon contained a higher amount of toxins than salmon caught in the wild (*Science*, 2004). The farmed salmon contained unusually high amounts of chemicals, pesticides, and potentially cancer-causing compounds called polychlorinated biphenyls (PCBs). We recommend to our patients that they ask specifically at the grocery store where the salmon was raised, as well as looking at the color of the fish. Wild-caught salmon is usually a brighter and/or deeper shade of pink or red, rather than the lighter shade of pink found in farm-raised varieties. Wild salmon is usually more expensive.

Lean Red Meat

Red meat has endured ups and downs in terms of its popularity and criticism in the media and also in nutrition circles. However, *lean* red meat in moderation can be an outstanding source of high-quality protein, as well as several vitamins and minerals. The key is to choose lean cuts (and opt for grass-fed, if possible). It is also important to trim the visible fat! Understanding the negative health effects, it makes us cringe to see people swallowing big bites of grizzly fat! Aside from the unnatural texture, it is objectively a squishy mouthful of "badness" for the body and brain.

LEANEST CUTS OF RED MEAT*

- Chuck Shoulder Steak
- Chuck Shoulder Pot Roast
- Shank Cross Cuts
- Round Steak
- Round Tip Roast and Steak
- Brisket, Flat Half
- Top Sirloin Steak
- Bottom Round Roast and Steak
- Top Round Roast and Steak
- Sirloin Tip Side Steak
- Eye Round Roast and Steak

*All have less than 175 calories, less than 7 grams total fat, and less than 2 grams saturated fat per 3-ounce serving, with visible fat trimmed.

FOODS WITH HIGH CONCENTRATIONS OF BOTH PROTEIN AND FAT

Red Meat

Although there are twenty-nine cuts of red meat that the USDA considers lean (less than 10 grams of total fat, 4.5 grams of saturated fat, and 95 mg of cholesterol per 3-ounce serving), there are many more cuts that are not. Some of the worst offenders are rib-eye, T-bone, New York strip, porterhouse, and skirt. Just for comparison sake, 100 grams (3.5 ounces) of rib-eye steak (e.g., prime rib) delivers a whopping 466 calories, 38 grams total fat, and 15 grams saturated fat versus the same 100 grams of sirloin tip side steak, which delivers only 206 calories, 5 gram total fat, and 2 grams saturated fat. That is twice the calories and *seven* times as much saturated and total fat!

Pork

As much as the pork industry would like us to believe, pork is nowhere near as healthy as chicken. Even the leanest cuts of pork typically carry more saturated fat and calories than even dark-meat chicken or turkey. If you eat pork, eat it in moderation.

Dairy

There is quite a bit of debate about whether the human digestive system was designed to process dairy products. The evidence is not clear so we are not going to cover that debate here. However, we do want to warn that regular dairy products (not reduced fat or fat free) typically contain a large amount of saturated fat. A few common examples are provided below.

ITEM	SERVING SIZE	CAL	TOTAL FAT	SATURATED FAT
Whole milk	1 cup	146	8 g	5 g
Yogurt	1 cup	149	8 g	5 g
Cheddar cheese	1 cup (diced)	532	44 g	28 g

For anyone who loves everything on that list, there is good news: there are low-fat options for all of them. In fact, there are low-fat options for just about everything! As discussed, just be sure to check the sugar (especially) and sodium content in any low-fat foods purchased. Again, for those who insist that low-fat foods taste terrible, there is scientific evidence showing that most people cannot tell the difference. That means that most people, most of the time, for most things, cannot tell the difference between full-fat and low-fat versions!

Fast Foods

We hope it is pretty clear that most fast food is bad for one's body and brain. It can be *very* bad, and, in many circumstances, we do not recommend eating it unless absolutely necessary (e.g., after being lost in the desert for three days and it is the only thing available). This is not to say that certain fast-food chains do not have healthy options. Subway, for example, is known to offer several healthy options that can be relatively brain-healthy as well, although the bread will provide a good number of carbohydrates. Healthy options at fast-food restaurants are, however, a relatively rare exception to the rule. In fact, the meals offered at most regular restaurants fit this description. After reading this book, making brain healthier choices should be easier in restaurants of all types. We will discuss restaurant eating in greater detail later in Chapter 19.

Nuts and Peanuts

Although nuts are relatively high in fat, it is typically unsaturated (less bad) fat, but not all nuts are created equal either. Assuming they are dry roasted, 1 ounce of macadamia nuts have 200 calories, 21 grams total fat, and 3 grams saturated fat, while the same 1 ounce of regular peanuts have 164 calories, 14 gram total fat, and 2 grams saturated fat. When it comes to nuts, eat in moderation and be sure to check nutrition labels to monitor nutrient contents and serving size.

CONCEPT 3: OVERCOMING CHALLENGES IN EATING HIGH-QUALITY LEAN PROTEIN

Particularly for people who lose weight when following the Alzheimer's Diet, sufficient protein is vital for healthy functioning of the body and brain. Below are common challenges to achieving this and suggestions for overcoming them.

"How do I know if I'm getting enough protein each day?"

We recommend 1 gram of protein for every kilogram (kg = 2.2 pounds) of body weight per day. That means a 180-pound person would want about 80 grams of protein, whereas a 110-pound individual would want about 50 grams protein.

"How do I get more lean protein in my diet?"

Meal replacements are a great way to get additional protein. Again, we always recommend that people get as much of their protein from regular foods as possible. However, for anyone who might find this challenging, we recommend protein supplementation, typically in the form of a shake (powder) or protein bar. Look for varieties high in whey protein, which may be preferable to soy protein, as discussed earlier.

"I'm vegan/vegetarian. How do I get enough protein?"

Spinach, soybeans, and soybean products (e.g., tempeh) provide high levels of high-quality protein, which means they are not deficient in any essential amino acids, as are many or most plant protein products. Quinoa is a little less common, but it is also an outstanding source of complete protein (plus fiber, phosphorous, and magnesium, and it is gluten-free). We recommend at least several servings of these complete protein products per day. Although not considered complete protein products, foods such as tofu, seitan (a wheat-gluten meat substitute, lentils, veggie burgers, veggie hotdogs, soymilk, and broccoli are typically high in protein as well.

CHAPTER 12

Antioxidants

Antioxidants may prove to be a very important part of brain-healthy diet. There are ongoing studies to determine the extent to which eating a diet rich in antioxidants is helpful for cognition. One particular study is looking at the combination of omega-3 fatty acids plus blueberry powder. The investigators will be capturing data on metabolic parameters, inflammation, and uptake of omega-3 fatty acids, as well as the effects on cognition.

Considering the risk-benefit ratio, we recommend antioxidant-rich foods as part of the Alzheimer's Diet. There are several antioxidant-rich foods aside from blueberries that we recommend, and these include several types of berries (e.g., raspberries, cranberries, acai, cherries, strawberries, blackberries, and elderberries). Other fruits like tomatoes (especially cooked), pomegranates, red grapes (and grape juice), oranges, grapefruits, and apples are also high in antioxidants. We suggest at least one to two servings of these antioxidant-rich foods per day.

Recent evidence published in the journal *Archives of Neurology* (2012) by Devore and colleagues provides strong evidence in support of regular intake of blueberries and strawberries. In this study, eating these two berries on a regular basis was found to delay cognitive decline for over two years! (Read an interview with Dr. Isaacson on the topic at: http://www.huffingtonpost.com/2012/04/26/cognitive-impairment-study-berries_n_1453557.html). This study was part of the Nurses' Health Study (for more information on this study, see Chapter 17).

Berries can help prevent brain aging and memory loss due to their high content of flavonoids, which are powerful antioxidants. More specifically, anthocyanidin components found 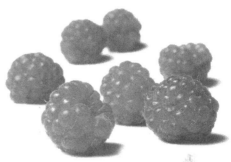 in high amounts in blueberries and strawberries can directly impact the memory centers in the brain. Other foods high in flavonoids (tea, dark chocolate, citrus fruits, and red wine) may also provide some benefit, but further studies are needed.

A variety of vegetables are high in antioxidants and other nutrients that may protect the brain. These include carrots, broccoli, beets, spinach, kale, cabbage, Brussels sprouts, artichokes, collard greens, and other dark leafy greens. Other high-antioxidant foods include walnuts, pecans, dark chocolate, tea (green and black), and coffee.

It is important to note that the jury is still out regarding the potential effects of antioxidants on memory function. As discussed in Chapter 6, a study in the journal *Archives of Neurology* in 2012 by Galasko and colleagues found that when taken in pill form, the antioxidant combination of vitamin E, C, and alpha-lipoic acid was found to have no effect on AD patients in a sixteen-week trial. Although spinal fluid lab markers slightly improved, memory function actually worsened slightly. In the same study, another antioxidant supplement called coenzyme Q10 also had no effect on memory function. However, while this study did not show benefit of these specific antioxidants via pill/supplement form, other studies have shown benefits of eating a diet rich in antioxidants and certain vitamins.

For the time being, many clinicians continue to recommend a diet rich in vitamins A and E, but do not routinely suggest that their patients take these vitamins, nor take alpha-lipoic acid or coenzyme Q10 in pill form.

A recent study in animals looked at the combination of a diet high in antioxidants together with behavioral enrichment. Researchers have studied these interventions in canines (beagles), since older animals develop a syndrome that is similar to Alzheimer's disease in humans. Dogs that develop cognitive deficits in middle age may be diagnosed with canine cognitive dysfunction Syndrome. Cognitive tests in dogs can be performed to help assess the effectiveness of an intervention, and their brains can be looked at under a microscope to determine if there are any effects apparent in the brain cells.

One study in canines looked at whether dietary antioxidants would reduce oxidative damage over three years. The antioxidant diet included added amounts of vitamin E and C, as well as spinach, carrots, tomatoes, citrus, grapes, lipoic acid, and l-carnitine (supplements that may help to protect the mitochondria, the cell's energy-producing centers). In addition to the enriched diet, dogs also participated in group exercise including three times per week of walking and running with other dogs (to incorporate socialization).

Dr. Carl Cotman and colleagues at the University of California at Irvine found that by the second year of the study, it was apparent that the intervention was working. By year three, the treatment group (diet and exercise) maintained cognition while almost 80 percent of the dogs that did not have the antioxidant-rich diet and exercise (control group) could no longer maintain the ability to perform specific cognitive tasks. In fact, over time, the diet and exercise group dogs regained the capacity to perform a task that they could do when they were younger. The control group dogs were unable to relearn the task. In addition, a study in the *Journal of Neuroscience* looked at amyloid protein load, which also decreased.

The take-home point here is that the combined treatment of an antioxidant-rich diet plus exercise led to improved brain function and better enabled protective mechanisms. While these studies need to be replicated in humans, it seems that exercise and behavioral enrichment work synergistically with diet to enhance brain health.

As such, in his clinical practice Dr. Isaacson advocates for combining brain-healthy dietary changes with exercise on a regular basis. Those patients that have done both together, as well as integrated socialization elements into their exercise routines, have in his clinical experience had the most significant positive benefits. "Social" aspects added to life in general as well as exercise may prove to be an important aspect toward maximizing brain health. Translating these research findings directly to humans is necessary and will take several years, but why wait? Considering the risk-benefit ratio, this combined effort is a strategy that Dr. Isaacson advocates for all of his patients.

CHAPTER 13

Caffeine/Coffee

There has been a lot of discussion in the media about whether caffeine and coffee should be considered in the treatment and/or prevention plans for Alzheimer's disease. This is due to several laboratory studies that show the potential for beneficial effects on brain health. While there are no scientific studies that specifically address caffeine and coffee as a treatment for AD, and while we also need more high-quality research in terms of prevention, we advocate for Mom's rule of "everything in moderation" when it comes to coffee and caffeine.

It should be okay to have 2 to 3 cups earlier in the day, but in the case of people with AD, this should first be approved by the treating physician. Drinking coffee after lunch is not recommended, as it may affect the sleep-wake cycle and impair a person's ability to effectively fall asleep (even up to ten hours after drinking it!). Also, caffeine may have effects on the heart (such as increasing heart rate) and may increase anxiety.

Studies done in Europe over several years demonstrate that men who drank coffee regularly for many years showed less of a decline on memory testing than did men who did not drink coffee. There was also a dose-related effect, meaning that the most benefit was in the group that drank three cups per day. Another study in France followed the coffee consumption of a group of men and women for four years. The results showed that women who were heavy drinkers (three or more 100-mg caffeine servings per day) showed less of a decline in verbal and visuospatial memory. However, there was no effect in men, and no impact on the emergence of dementia.

The most recent study in mice yielded some very interesting results. Cao and colleagues found that mice with (the mouse-version of) AD that drank the human equivalent of several cups of coffee each day had cognitive benefits (*Journal of Alzheimer's Disease*, June 2011). In addition, several other studies have shown the potential for a "protective" effect of caffeine/coffee on the brain. The theory behind this is that caffeine (or perhaps a yet unidentified substance in caffeinated coffee) may have a protective effect on the brain (perhaps by blocking the toxic effects of beta-amyloid). As such, coffee intake in moderation (as long as it is not late in the day) is one of the components of the Alzheimer's Diet.

CHAPTER 14

Dietary Ketosis—12-Hour Fast

The *Alzheimer's Diet* advocates for eating a lower amount of carbohydrates than is recommended by the United States Department of Agriculture (USDA), as long as this is approved and supervised by the treating physician. There are a variety of definitions used for what would be the amount of total carbohydrate grams per day to qualify for a low-carbohydrate diet. Some would say eating less than the Recommended Daily Allowance (RDA) amount of 130 g per day would qualify. Others would say less than 60 grams per day would qualify. In this book, at the end of the 9-week diet plan, we suggest eating about half of the RDA of 130 grams as a daily dietary goal. On the contrary, the definition of a *very* low carbohydrate is actually quite different than that of a low-carbohydrate diet. When a person eats less than 20–30 grams of carbohydrates each day, this can lead to a prolonged state of brain/body metabolism called ketosis. In this state, the body will produce substances called ketone bodies (which cause ketosis) that can be used as an alternative energy source for the brain. There is scientific evidence that ketone bodies may not only have a protective effect on the brain cells, but also improve memory function in patients with MCI or AD. This is most likely due to the fact that the brains of AD patients have a decreased ability to use glucose as a fuel, and the only alternative energy source that the brain can use is ketone bodies.

Despite this evidence, and for a variety of reasons, *The Alzheimer's Diet* does not suggest a very-low carbohydrate diet. First off, there can be negative health consequences in certain patients from prolonged ketosis. Secondly, compliance with a very low-carbohydrate diet is difficult, mostly related to the fact that is very challenging to eat such a small amount of carbohydrates in a day. In fact, most people who attempt a very low-carbohydrate diet are unable to adhere due to the sheer amount of carbohydrate restriction.

As a compromise, we suggest that patients decrease their carbohydrate intake over time, and also occasionally advocate for the "early-bird special" technique when it comes to dietary modification. The early-bird special is a special pricing deal at some restaurants when the diners are seated before 6 p.m. It turns out saving money isn't the only benefit here. There may also be a brain-boosting effect associated with early dinners.

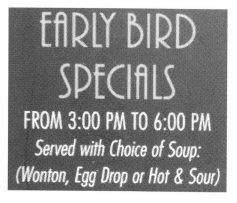

In some patients, waiting at least twelve hours between dinner and breakfast can bring about a very mild state of ketosis. This technique, combined with minimal (if any) carbohydrates in the morning, requires further research but may make sense from a brain/body metabolism perspective. Remember, there is some evidence that a state of ketosis may have "anti-aging" effects on the brain. As such, even trying this approach several days a week may be a reasonable option to reduce risk, but only when approved by one's primary-care physician. Of course, this means no late-night snacking between dinner and breakfast!

A variety of scientific studies have evaluated the effect of ketosis on brain health and several have found positive results. Aside from the 12-hour fast described above and aside from following a very low-carbohydrate diet, there are other ways to achieve ketosis that we will discuss below.

Any efforts at achieving ketosis must be approved and supervised by the treating physician. Great care must be taken to avoid negative or severe health consequences—for example, certain people with diabetes (usually type 1 but also type 2) may be at risk of the dangerous condition called diabetic ketoacidosis. Therefore, such patients would be advised to avoid very low or no carbohydrate diets.

In Chapter 23, we discuss an FDA-regulated medical food that has been studied in the treatment of AD. This product contains a medium chain triglyceride (MCT) called caprylic triglyceride (trade name Axona), which has been shown to provide cognitive benefits for patients with mild to moderate AD who are negative for the APOE4 gene. (See Chapter 15 for more details on how a person's genes play a role in his or her likelihood to respond to a therapeutic agent.) Caprylic triglyceride (Axona) is predominantly converted to the ketone body beta-hydroxybutyrate in the liver, and this then circulates to the brain and can be used as a fuel. This therapy is currently available by prescription.

As discussed in Chapter 8, AD can be studied in animals, specifically dogs, as they have similar characteristic proteins found in humans with AD (beta-amyloid). A research study published in 2008 in the journal *Brain Research* by Studzinski and colleagues examined the effects on giving the main ingredient in Axona (caprylic triglyceride) to aged beagles. This led to lower levels of oxidative damage found in the mitochondria, which suggests that there may be some protective mechanism on brain function. Further studies in humans are warranted and necessary to clarify these results and to determine effectiveness on brain protection.

In Chapter 17, we review the background on using coconut oil, which is also a medium-chain triglyceride (MCT). MCTs are converted to ketone bodies in the liver and, as mentioned above, can be used in the brain as an alternative fuel source. There are limited data evaluating the effectiveness of coconut oil, and further study is warranted on this therapeutic strategy for AD treatment and prevention. Risks/benefits of coconut oil also need to be discussed in detail with the treating physician, since there is the potential for adverse effects. These are discussed later on in Chapter 17 in greater detail.

CHAPTER 15

Nutrigenomics: The Effects of Genetics on the Effectiveness of Dietary Interventions

Nutrigenomics is a field of science that studies the relationship between food intake and the expression of one's genes. To clarify, nutrigenomics arose from the observation that each individual, depending on their genetic code, responds differently to specific dietary intakes. This field is an area that will likely expand a great deal in the coming years.

The term "nutrigenomics" is similar to the term "pharmacogenomics," which refers to certain interventions that may preferentially work in certain individuals (who have or do not have specific genes). For example, in certain studies, people without a specific gene (APOE4) responded better to therapies like DHA fish oil (for the treatment of age-associated cognitive decline) and the medical food Axona (for patients with Alzheimer's disease).

Further scientific study is necessary, and future results should promote a broader understanding of how nutrition influences cellular function and metabolic pathways. This, in turn, can then be used to delay or even possibly prevent certain chronic disease that may come about due to poor dietary choices over time. Aside from Alzheimer's disease and general cognitive decline, other common conditions like metabolic syndrome, obesity, diabetes, and heart disease may be closely tied to dietary consumption. Isolating specific genes in an effort to further understand the effect of these assorted genetic predispositions may help clinicians in the future to advise patients on which foods to avoid and which to maximize. It is likely that personalized dietary recommendations will be given with increasing frequency as the science evolves.

CHAPTER 16

Multicultural Considerations

Current research suggests that the incidence of Alzheimer's disease or cognitive impairment affects certain ethnicities more so than others. This may be due to a combination of factors, such as genetics, diet patterns, or the interaction of both of these (as discussed in the previous chapter). In addition, there are many medical problems, including diabetes and high blood pressure, that are found more frequently in certain ethnicities, especially Hispanic-Americans and African-Americans. These medical conditions may increase the likelihood of developing AD, lead to worsening of AD symptoms, or lead to an earlier onset of memory loss. Optimizing diet and nutrition is especially important in anyone with these diagnoses.

The Alzheimer's Association compiled two separate comprehensive reports that both concluded that AD is more common in African-Americans and Hispanic-Americans (see the websites listed at the end of this chapter). For example, in African-Americans, estimates range from an incidence of 14 percent to almost 100 percent greater; again, this may due to a combination of factors.

A growing body of evidence indicates that medical conditions like diabetes is a strong risk factor for AD, in part due to the negative effects on blood vessels over time (which in turn lead to damaged brain cells). For example, Hispanic-Americans have a 64 percent higher risk of diabetes than non-Hispanic white Americans. A study of older Mexican-Americans found that type 2 diabetes and high blood pressure contribute more to dementia in this ethnic group than in people of European ancestry.

A recent study published in the *British Medical Journal* (2011) by Adelman and colleagues found that African-Caribbeans living in England had a higher likelihood of developing dementia. The results found that the prevalence of dementia was significantly higher in African-Caribbeans compared to whites (9.6 percent vs. 6.9 percent), and that people of African-Caribbean descent with dementia were nearly eight years younger than those in the white group (after correcting for age and socioeconomic status).

Similarly, a study by Clark and colleagues found that Hispanic-Americans develop AD 6.8 years earlier than their white, non-Hispanic peers (2004). Further studies are necessary to determine the reasons behind this increased risk.

An article published by Jones and colleagues in the *Journal of Aging Studies* used ten focus groups from Asian-American communities representing different national origins (including Chinese, Japanese, and Korean) to examine factors shaping attitudes toward AD. Attitudes toward barriers to timely diagnosis and treatment were also studied. Results suggested that while these communities had strong awareness of AD, beliefs may be influenced at least as strongly by folk wisdom and culturally acceptable partial truths as by scientific information (2006). Similar findings have been found in other ethnic groups as well.

MULTICULTURAL CONSIDERATION FOR DIET AND NUTRITION: DIET IN GENERAL VERSUS NUTRIGENOMICS

Notions of what constitutes a healthy diet vary between ethnicities and cultures. The dietary interventions in this book are designed to be maximally beneficial for preserving brain function in all ethnicities. Remember, we are not concerned with body shape or weight or even different kinds of foods. The goal of these changes is not to "lose those love handles," but to preserve memory and other cognitive functions. We prefer that people think of these dietary modifications as making brain-healthy changes in their diet, rather than as "going on" a brain-healthy diet. In the future, the medical community will learn more about the influence of ethnicity (and more specifically, a person's genes) on how the body responds to the food choices they make. The area of personalized nutrition will likely expand rapidly and apply differently to those of different races or ethnicities. Further study is warranted regarding the exciting area of nutrigenomics.

For more information on the Alzheimer's Association reports mentioned above, visit:

http://www.alz.org/national/documents/latino_brochure_ diabetes.pdf

http://www.alz.org/alzwa/documents/alzwa_resource_cult_ hispanicreportenglish.pdf

http://www.alz.org/national/documents/report_african americanssilentepidemic.pdf

http://www.alz.org/national/documents/minorities_ english.pdf

CHAPTER 17

The Future of AD Diet Research

There has been an explosion of research in the area of nutrition and AD. For the first time in 2011, the International Clinical Trials in Alzheimer's Disease Conference added "Nutrition" to their presentation research category. In 2012, the number of research projects in that category increased by over 400 percent (representing nearly 10 percent of all research presented)! A myriad of investigators from all over the world are now embarking on the next frontier of AD nutrition research and innovation.

DR. ISAACSON:

There is a natural progression that occurs within science over time. With every passing week it seems that there is more and more evidence for diet and its influence on the brain and AD. Unfortunately, many physicians, patients, and caregivers are still in the dark about these research findings.

As an AD specialist with several family members affected, I tend to look quite differently at this disease. Based on my family history, I try to keep ahead of the curve when it comes to such evidence. Two years ago, I had a conversation with a colleague considered to be a national leader in Alzheimer's disease. He asked me directly, "Is there really any convincing evidence that diet changes can help with Alzheimer's treatment or prevention?" As academic neurologists often do, I spouted off a number of what I consider to be very convincing studies on diet and AD. I stated the journal and author names, dates, titles of the studies, and a summary of the results. I was surprised that my colleague was unaware of this exciting progress, but as he later explained, he had been most recently spending his time in the research lab, and had not been caring for patients in his clinic for quite some time.

Fast-forward the clock a few years, and it is now common knowledge among most experts (including my aforementioned colleague!) that dietary changes are a strong and necessary intervention for both treatment and prevention.

PREDICTIONS FOR THE FUTURE

So, where do we go from here and what does the future hold for diet and AD? For centuries, scholars have suggested specific dietary recommendations, and yet we have only recently begun to expand the scientific evidence behind their wisdom. For example, "Hara hachi bu" is a Confucian teaching that suggests people should only eat until they are roughly 80 percent full (translated from Japanese). Confucius (551–478 BC) was a Chinese philosopher who developed a philosophical system that even included dietary suggestions. Today, in the city of Okinawa, Japan, this practice of self-imposed calorie restriction has led to nearly *30 percent* of citizens living to the age of 100 (almost four times the average in Western countries like the United States!).

CALORIC RESTRICTION

In the area of AD, mild cognitive impairment (MCI) and cognitive impairment in general, more research is necessary on how caloric restriction can help to prevent or delay the onset of AD or cognitive decline. In 2012, Geda and colleagues released their findings from the Mayo Clinic Study of Aging that found overeating could double the risk of memory loss. This study found that eating more (versus less) than 2,142 calories per day was associated with significantly increased odds of having MCI.

BERRY GOOD NEWS! MORE EVIDENCE FOR DIETARY ANTIOXIDANTS FOR AD

As discussed earlier, strong evidence supports that regular intake of blueberries and strawberries can delay cognitive decline for over two years! (Read an interview with Dr. Isaacson on this topic at: http://www.huffingtonpost.com/2012/04/26/cognitive-impairment-study-berries_n_1453557.html). This study was part of the well-known Nurses' Health Study (among the most well-structured and longest-running research studies examining women's health in the United States). As Dr. Isaacson says in the interview, if you can delay the onset of cognitive decline by six months (let alone two or more years), the impact on individual health, as well as the overall health of our society, would be immeasurable.

How can berries help to prevent brain aging and memory loss? Flavonoids (an antioxidant), or more specifically anthocyanidin components, which are found in high amounts in blueberries and strawberries, can directly impact the memory centers in the brain. Other foods high in flavonoids may also help (tea, dark chocolate, citrus fruits, and red wine), but further study is necessary and should include different demographic groups (e.g., men) as well. The study was published in the journal *Archives of Neurology* by Devore and colleagues (affiliated with Harvard Medical School).

While these findings are exciting, more studies are needed to determine whether these types of berries could have a benefit for treating AD. More research will also clarify the cognitive benefits of eating berries when used in combination with the other diet strategies detailed in this book. Currently, it is difficult to know how long a person needs to eat flavonoid-rich foods to protect the brain. Regardless, dietary changes made today will likely lead to incremental changes of brain functioning over time.

Other recent research by Scarmeas and colleagues at Columbia University College of Physicians and Surgeons has found that the Mediterranean diet (which is high in antioxidants) reduces the risk of cognitive decline and MCI. For example, one study found that the Mediterranean diet was associated with a trend for reduced risk of developing MCI and also with a reduced risk of MCI converting to AD.

The Mediterranean diet (see Chapter 14 for more information) is generally composed of 25 percent to 35 percent of calories from fat, but with less than 8 percent of saturated fat. Olive oil (extra-virgin) is most characteristic, as it is made up of very high levels of certain monounsaturated fats (oleic acid), which research studies have shown to be protective for conditions like heart disease. Antioxidants in olive oil may also help reduce inflammation, blood pressure, and LDL cholesterol ("bad" cholesterol), as well as help with overall cholesterol regulation.

Dr. Walter Willett, Professor of Medicine at Harvard Medical School, was one of the most prominent physicians to help popularize the Mediterranean diet, and there has been much interest in this style of eating for several reasons. In the late 1950s, Dr. Ancel Keys from the University of Minnesota devised the Seven Countries Study. This study demonstrated that, as people living in the Mediterranean region shifted from a healthy diet and active lifestyle to a less active lifestyle and more of a "Western" diet, risk of heart disease increased dramatically. Several other studies have been published since, including one from the *British Medical Journal* (2008) that revealed that following strictly the Mediterranean diet reduced the risk of developing not only AD, but also Parkinson's disease, and the risk of dying from cancer and heart disease as well.

CHOLESTEROL AND AD

Another area that warrants further study is the effect of cholesterol levels and efforts to reduce blood levels of cholesterol on the development of cognitive decline and AD, as well as for AD treatment. Most will agree that ongoing follow-up with a primary-care physician (e.g., internist or family practice doctor) is imperative for routine health maintenance. Treating physicians can discuss with their patients a number of ways to reduce cholesterol (e.g., diet, other lifestyle changes, medication). Physicians also pay close attention to vascular risk factors (cholesterol, high blood pressure, diabetes, high blood sugar), which have the potential to increase the rate of progression of memory decline. Individuals should have cholesterol results checked on a regular basis and consider treatment if levels are abnormal. In addition to diet modification, cholesterol drugs may benefit patients with high cholesterol (the most commonly used medications are called statins). A recent study by Sano and colleagues in mild to moderate AD patients with normal cholesterol failed to show benefit of disease progression (*Neurology*, 2011) when treated with a statin drug called simvastatin. The risks and benefits of statin use should be discussed in detail with the physician and further studies in the future may help to clarify which statin drugs, if any, may yield either a treatment or preventative effect on AD.

CONTROVERSIES IN THE CONNECTION BETWEEN CHOLESTEROL AND AD

An article published last year by Seneff and colleagues (*European Journal of Internal Medicine*) details a comprehensive review of nutrition and AD, including the detrimental role of a high-carbohydrate diet. This article describes research evidence suggesting that a defect in cholesterol metabolism in the brain may play an important role in AD. About fifteen years ago, Notkola and colleagues studied whether high cholesterol levels might actually be an attempt on the part of the body to "adjust" for a poor rate of cholesterol uptake in the brain. Their findings were published in the journal *Neuroepidemiology*, and found that in a group of men aged seventy to eighty-nine, cholesterol levels fell for those who developed AD prior to their showing AD symptoms. The authors suggested high cholesterol could have been a protective mechanism against AD. Other studies have found that higher cholesterol levels correlated with increased life span in those over eighty-five years of age, and have also been associated with better memory function and reduced rates of dementia. Further study is warranted. In the meantime, most clinicians continue to recommend treating high cholesterol levels, especially with the significant protective evidence on heart disease, vascular disease, and stroke.

COCONUT OIL

There has been recent attention given to the possibility of using coconut oil for AD prevention and treatment. A significant amount of research is needed in order to clarify which types of coconut oil may work best, as well as positive and negative outcomes (if any) on both cognitive measures and other health markers (e.g., body weight, cholesterol).

There are several reasons coconut oil has received attention in the management of AD. Coconut oil is made up of medium chain triglycerides (or MCTs), which can be used as an alternative fuel source in the brain, and may have protective qualities against brain aging. MCTs are broken down by the liver to form ketone bodies, which is the only fuel the brain can utilize aside from sugar.

Without sufficient scientific research, many physicians have not yet recommended coconut oil for widespread use in their AD patients. Some physicians are cautious since certain types of coconut oils can actually raise cholesterol and may have harmful effects when used in large amounts. Those physicians who suggest coconut oil advocate for using only particular types, specifically non-hydrogenated without any trans fats. The hydrogenated forms of coconut oil can raise cholesterol and should be avoided.

Due to the high-fat content in coconut oil, there is the possibility of gaining weight if too much is eaten. As such, it is important to reduce other fat intake in meals in a complementary fashion. Reducing portion sizes, selecting non-fat or low-fat foods, and making sure to stick to an active exercise regimen will be important if making the decision to try coconut oil for AD treatment or prevention. Additionally, any and all changes need to be made under the guidance and supervision of the treating physician. Weight and lab tests (e.g., cholesterol levels) should be monitored as well.

A rule of thumb when it comes to coconut oil is that, if it is started, it should be started in very small amounts and increased slowly and gradually over time. Side effects such as diarrhea, stomach cramping, bloating, nausea, or vomiting can occur, especially if started too quickly. Individuals with a history of bleeding in the gastrointestinal tract, inflammatory diseases of the gastrointestinal tract, and a variety of other medical conditions need to be very cautious with the use of coconut oil.

Until further research is done, we are not sure whether to advocate for the use of coconut or MCT oil in our patients, and thus have not yet begun to routinely recommend it. However, we also do not strongly suggest against our patients trying it (as long as they remain mindful of the amount of saturated fat and potential for adverse effects as described above).

For those individuals already taking coconut or MCT oil, or those who under physician supervision decide to try it, it is not yet known how much would be optimal for brain health.

One method that has been tried by clinicians is starting with a half of a teaspoon with a meal for a few days, then increasing to a full teaspoon with a meal for a few days, and slowly increasing to 1 teaspoon twice per day after a week. If tolerated and approved by the treating physician, this may be slowly increased over time to 1–2 tablespoons with meals (two or three times a day). Different brands of coconut oil provide different amounts of MCTs, and it is unclear which brands might work better (or at all) since they have not been individually studied and are not regulated by the FDA. Further research is warranted to determine whether coconut oil is effective for the prevention or treatment of AD and, if so, to clarify which patient types (e.g., genetics) and which stages of AD (e.g., pre-Alzheimer's, MCI) are best suited to respond. For those interested in the potential of using MCTs to enhance brain function and improve memory in patients with AD, read more about the medical food Axona (caprylic triglyceride) in Chapter 23.

GLUTEN AND ALZHEIMER'S DISEASE

Is there a relationship between gluten intake and AD or cognitive impairment? Before we discuss this further, it is important to review a few introductory points.

BACKGROUND ON GLUTEN

The word "gluten" is derived from Latin (meaning *glue*) and refers to the protein component that keeps wheat "stuck together." Wheat is a type of grain (from which flour is made). This flour is then used to make a variety of foods, like bread, pasta, and cake. Wheat gluten is found in many different types of food, including breakfast cereals, beer, crackers, soy sauce, and some preparations of ketchup.

Many of the most common types of grain contain gluten. These include barley, rye, bulgur, and as mentioned earlier, wheat. Other types of grains that do not contain gluten include rice, wild rice, and buckwheat (or kasha).

While certain types of grains may be "gluten-free" by composition, it is important to note that there may be a chance that these grains are handled or processed in an environment where cross contamination with gluten is a possibility. Therefore, if a person has a gluten allergy or intolerance (more on these conditions later), they must be very careful and pay close attention when selecting grains to eat.

Quinoa, while often thought to be a grain, is actually a seed that is considered "grain-like." It is gluten-free and rich in high-quality protein. Millet is a grain that looks like quinoa and is also gluten-free. Millet looks similar to couscous; however, couscous is a pasta not a grain, thus it contains gluten.

FAST FACTS ABOUT GRAINS:

- Barley: High in fiber and can help lower cholesterol.

- Bulgur: Less fat and more fiber than brown rice, with the same amount of protein. Also a good source of potassium, B vitamins, iron, and calcium.

- Buckwheat: High in fiber, B vitamins, and helpful for stabilizing blood sugar. Contains eight essential amino acids and may also lower blood pressure and cholesterol.

- Kasha (or roasted buckwheat): High in protein, fiber, and antioxidants. May also help lower blood pressure and cholesterol.

- Millet: Contains protein and high amounts of fiber, B vitamins, and the minerals iron, magnesium, phosphorous, and potassium.

You have probably read the term "whole grain" on food packages. Whole grain is defined as containing all of the naturally occurring elements of the grain, such as the bran, endosperm (e.g., starchy carbohydrates, protein) and germ. You may also have seen the term "whole wheat," which is a form of whole grain. Wheat is just one type of grain. The important thing is to look for "whole" on the packaging (or first ingredient), and avoid "multigrain" or "seven-grain," as these may still not contain the healthiest parts of the grains.

GLUTEN INTOLERANCE

Up to 1 percent of people in the United States have a gluten-sensitivity due to celiac disease. This is a medical condition that is characterized by an abnormal immune reaction when gluten is consumed. This reaction can cause a variety of symptoms, such as stomach pain, bloating, diarrhea, weakness, fatigue, and weight loss.

A wheat allergy is different from celiac disease and is actually an allergic reaction to foods containing wheat. The most common types of food allergies include peanuts, tree nuts (hazelnuts and almonds), milk, eggs, fish, and several types of shellfish (shrimp, lobster, and crab). When a person with a food allergy eats that specific food, urgent medical attention may need to be sought, since medication may be needed to prevent serious health consequences (for example, breathing trouble and closing of the airways, which could lead to death).

A wheat allergy causes the body to release an allergy-causing particle (antibody) to the proteins that are found in wheat. The specific protein gluten is the culprit here, since it causes an abnormal immune system response in the digestive tract (small intestine) of people with celiac disease.

RESEARCH ON CELIAC DISEASE AND COGNITIVE IMPAIRMENT

In 2006, a study was published in the journal *Archives of Neurology* by Hu and colleagues at Mayo Clinic that examined the relationship between celiac disease and cognitive impairment. A diagnosis of celiac disease had to be proven by a biopsy, or tissue sample. While only thirteen patients were studied, there seemed to be a possible association between decline in thinking skills and celiac disease. Three of these patients improved or stabilized cognitively when they stopped eating gluten. To truly identify a cause-and-effect relationship, further study is necessary to clarify this relationship, as the number of patients included in the study was small, and a more scientifically rigorous approach in the future may yield results that will be easier to interpret (of note, this group did not include any patients with a diagnosis of AD).

RESEARCH ON CELIAC DISEASE AND AD

There is limited data on the relationship between celiac disease and AD. One study in 2008 by Bodil Roth and colleagues in the *Scandinavian Journal of Immunology* failed to find an association between antibodies related to celiac disease in patients with AD. Another study also published in 2008 by Lurie and colleagues in the *Journal of Clinical Gastroenterology* examined the medical charts of seven patients diagnosed with celiac disease after the age of sixty. Two female patients presented with cognitive decline that was attributed to AD, but improved after starting a gluten-free diet. This suggests that further study is warranted.

RELATIONSHIP OF GLUTEN TO COGNITIVE IMPAIRMENT AND AD

As mentioned, high amounts of carbohydrates in the diet may be related to an increased risk of AD, and decreasing carbs significantly can lead to improved memory (according to test scores based on several research studies). Therefore, gluten reduction may indirectly protect the brain, as people who reduce or eliminate gluten from their diet may also be reducing overall carbohydrate intake. However, while this may be true for some with gluten intolerance, there is much variability with carbohydrate intake. It is not a generalizable concept, especially with the increase in gluten-free products available for widespread purchase that are high in fat, added sugar, and other high-glycemic carbohydrates).

But does gluten itself cause Alzheimer's or make AD symptoms worse? At the time of publication of this book, there is no scientific evidence that supports this. The answer to this question may depend on a variety of factors, and more research will be needed to clarify this. If you are sensitive to gluten, or have celiac disease, antibodies in the intestines will react to the gluten protein and cause a cascade of events, such as the release of inflammatory markers (e.g., cytokines), interaction with specific genes (or in other words turning a gene "on" or "off") or combining directly with certain proteins found in the brain. Any of these interactions could potentially have a detrimental effect on brain function and, as an example, scientists believe that inflammation in the brain can be related to the development or worsening of AD symptoms.

As an analogy, think about what happens when a person falls and sprains his or her ankle. The ankle joint becomes inflamed and swells. A similar type of inflammation can happen in the brain and, just as it is difficult to walk after an ankle injury, the brain will have a harder time functioning in terms of thinking skills and memory.

When it comes to the effect of gluten on the brain, research has shown that people with gluten sensitivity can develop negative neurological outcomes. A study in the journal *Pediatrics* (Zelnik and colleagues) in 2004 described a broader variability of neurologic disorders that occur in celiac disease than previously recognized, including attention deficit/hyperactivity disorder (ADHD), developmental delay, chronic headache, and even learning disorders. Additional research has associated gluten intolerance and intake with a number of other non-neurological conditions in children, including infectious diseases (e.g., ear infections, bronchitis), inflammatory/allergic conditions (e.g., skin rash), and behavioral abnormalities (e.g., low energy, moodiness).

Additional scientific research will help to clarify the differences between negative health effect of gluten for those individuals with and without gluten sensitivity. As touched upon in the chapter on nutrigenomics, a one-size-fits-all approach to dietary and nutrition management may not apply considering these individualized aspects.

FOOD ALLERGIES

When making changes to the diet, there is the potential of trying new foods that have not been tried in the past. For this reason, this section will briefly review food allergies. Regardless of one's health status, it is essential to seek an evaluation by a physician if a food allergy or food intolerance is suspected. In addition to asking a series of questions and collecting information about the nature of the problem (e.g., food diary, family history), a physician may order lab tests (a blood test or a skin prick test for a food allergy), or even a diagnostic procedure if celiac disease is suspected (e.g., a tissue biopsy performed by a gastroenterologist).

For food allergies, a blood test will look for different amounts of food-specific antibodies that may be present. The skin prick test requires the injection of a small amount of food extract (or a needle that was soaked in the food extract is used) to determine if there is a skin reaction (a "mosquito-bite"-type mark at the injection site).

For example, in the case of celiac disease, there are blood tests that can help with diagnosis, but these tests are not perfect. Therefore, positive results on a blood test may require additional testing (biopsy from the small intestine).

Remember that food allergy and intolerance testing are helpful in identifying (or excluding) a food allergy or intolerance as a cause of symptoms. However, there is a great deal of complexity behind selecting which tests should be ordered and subsequently understanding how the results should be interpreted. For more information on food allergy testing, visit the Food Allergy & Anaphylaxis Network's website: www.foodallergy.org.

Since eliminating certain foods from the diet or reintroducing other foods back to the diet can lead to serious negative medical/health consequences, the supervising physician should be consulted every time a change is made. For severe allergic reactions, emergency medical attention may be necessary, as an emergency injection of the drug epinephrine may be necessary. Always seek the help of a qualified medical professional and call 911 or visit the closest emergency room for such events. In order to minimize risk of an allergic reaction, always carefully read the nutritional label and ingredient list. When in doubt, do not eat something that is potentially harmful. This is especially true at parties, social events, and restaurants, since even a very small amount of a food can cause a severe allergic reaction.

ALCOHOL

The effect of alcohol consumption on AD prevention is currently unclear. Data suggests that one serving (in women) or one to two servings (in men) per day may be reasonable to minimize the likelihood of developing AD. A recent article by Neafsey and Collins concluded that this amount may reduce the risk of dementia and cognitive decline (*Neuropsychiatric Disease and Treatment*, 2011), although further study is warranted. In terms of treatment, there is no evidence that alcohol helps memory and too much can certainly make it worse. Most physicians generally permit patients with AD to have small amounts of alcohol (e.g., a glass of wine with dinner), as long as these amounts do not negatively affect thinking skills or behavior. We advise against consumption of more than one or two servings per day in our patients, as this may lead to negative health consequences.

Snapshots

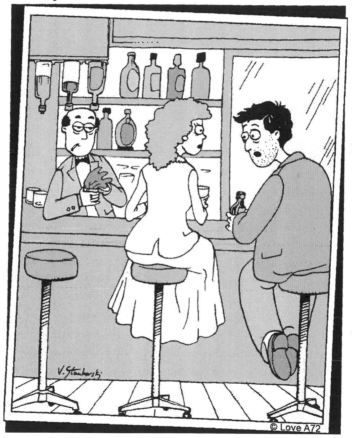

"I have a terrible memory. Do I come here often?"

SECTION 3:

WHAT SHOULD I EAT?

CHAPTER 18

Dietary Strategies and the 9-Week Diet Plan

T his chapter puts into action the dietary concepts we have been discussing throughout the first two sections of this book. The first part of this chapter provides general strategies for brain-healthy eating. The second part outlines the structured weekly plan for getting started on the Alzheimer's Diet.

> **IMPORTANT: All dietary changes should be made with the approval and under the guidance of the treating physician.** We also recommend consultation with a registered dietician to assist in adopting this plan.

PART ONE—DIETARY STRATEGIES

Individuals should be encouraged to utilize a combination of a brain-healthy diet and regular physical exercise. As discussed in Chapter 8, these can work synergistically to optimize health in fighting Alzheimer's disease. There are a variety of components of the 9-week plan; however, among the most essential are making these changes gradually, sustaining these changes over time, and adhering to a reduction of total carbohydrate intake (most specifically, the "bad" carbs). Note that based on the United States Department of Agriculture (USDA) Dietary Reference Intake report, the Recommended Daily Allowance (RDA) of carbohydrates is 130 grams per day (not including fiber). The Alzheimer's Diet plan outlined below will help guide the incremental decrease of carbohydrates, while also focusing on other changes based on scientific evidence.

We provide recommendations using grams of carbohydrates rather than percent of caloric intake, as this is easier to follow for most individuals. However, the actual number of grams of carbohydrates in a "low-carbohydrate" diet may vary depending on the total daily caloric intake of different individuals. For example, a petit female may only consume 1,800 calories per day to maintain her current body weight, while an obese male may consume 3,600 calories per day to maintain his current body weight. If both of these individuals consume the same number of grams of carbohydrates in a given day, the percentage of total calories ingested from carbohydrates in that day will be twice as high for the female versus the male, since she only consumes half the total number of calories.

Therefore, it is important to note that the target carbohydrate intake recommendations in the 9-Week Diet Plan are not based on caloric intake per se, but instead are based on our clinical experience with asking our patients to choose an attainable goal of carbohydrate restriction. Highly active individuals (like athletes) and those who are obese may wish to adjust their target carbohydrate upward to account for the fact that they consume more calories. However, we do not recommend adjusting target carbohydrate intake below that recommended in the 9-Week Diet Plan without prior approval and strict supervision by a physician. It is also important to note that medical research has not yet established precise guidelines for brain-healthy total carbohydrate intake, either in number of grams or percentage of total caloric intake. Therefore, the recommendations provided in the 9-Week Diet Plan are the best estimates that can be provided based on the available scientific data.

DR. ISAACSON:

One story that I like to share is from my earlier years as a treating physician. I spoke with a nutritional scientist who also has a strong family history of Alzheimer's disease. I asked him the following question: What is the number-one thing that you would suggest to potentially delay the onset of Alzheimer's? His response was simple—a low-carbohydrate diet, avoiding simple sugars. I have since adopted these changes in my own life to help reduce my own risk for AD, and I recommended these strategies to countless patients and their family members. Through the years, I have expanded and honed this strategy based on my own experience as well as the experience of my patients. In this section, I give "real-life" examples of my personal decisions regarding food choices that may reduce the risk of developing AD.

Let's review the essential nutritional aspects for attempting to delay the onset of, or treat, Alzheimer's. As discussed earlier, the three different types of macronutrients are proteins, fats, and carbohydrates. The following are rules of thumb for macronutrient consumption:

MAXIMIZE:

- High-quality lean protein. Examples of recommended protein sources include fish high in DHA (e.g., wild salmon, mackerel, lake trout, herring, sardines, albacore tuna), poultry (skinless white-meat chicken and turkey), and lean meats (beef), which are hormone free when possible, egg whites, and low- or non-fat dairy products.

- Vegetables (especially dark-green leafy vegetables) and berries (especially strawberries and blueberries). Note that these healthy choices do contain low-glycemic (good) carbohydrates that should be tracked.

EAT IN MODERATION:

- Monounsaturated (e.g., extra-virgin olive oil, peanuts, avocados) and polyunsaturated fats (e.g., nuts and seeds).

- Complex carbohydrates (e.g., whole grains, quinoa)

MINIMIZE:

- Simple (high-glycemic) carbohydrates (e.g., white bread, cane sugar, high fructose corn syrup, and corn syrup in general)

- Saturated fats (eliminate trans fats)

From our discussions on the importance of insulin, it should be clear why minimizing simple, or high-glycemic, carbohydrates is a sensible idea. Simple carbohydrates are composed of a single sugar molecule or two joined sugar molecules, such as glucose, fructose, lactose, and sucrose. In addition to the examples given earlier, simple carbohydrates also include brown sugar, fruit sugar, molasses, honey, and candy. Avoiding this type of sugar completely is very difficult, but not impossible. However, with dedication and education, many people have made constructive changes to their diets.

Overall, reducing added sugars and selecting complex carbohydrates (as opposed to simple carbohydrates) as part of a balanced diet is most important. Complex carbohydrates are defined as large chains of sugar units arranged to form starches and fiber. These include vegetables, whole fruits, grains (brown rice, buckwheat, quinoa, oats, wheat, barley, corn), and legumes (chickpeas, black-eyed peas, lentils, as well as beans such as lima, kidney, pinto, soy, and black beans). Sugary and starchy foods like pasta and white rice break down quickly to sugar and thus should be minimized. When selecting pasta in the grocery store, be sure to read the label closely. When possible, choose whole wheat and added protein varieties.

Dr. Isaacson:

When making changes to one's diet, old habits are hard to break. In my clinical practice, I insist that these dietary modifications are made slowly but surely, beginning as far as possible before the onset of AD symptoms, or soon after a diagnosis of AD.

Personally, I wind up skipping breakfast several times per week. I typically finish dinner by 7 p.m., so my next meal may not be until noon the following day. While the mild state of ketosis resulting from this "mini fast" may be protective for me, I am unsure of the exact benefit. Regardless, it is a strategy that has been approved by my own primary-care physician and fits with my lifestyle, work habits, and schedule. The scientific data on mini-fasts (e.g., skipping breakfast) is mixed; however, this strategy works for me in a few ways. It leads to my consuming fewer overall calories during the day and also fits with my personal preference of morning exercise (as exercise may have a greater benefit after a night of fasting, in that a person will burn most calories from fat instead of carbohydrates).

I minimize carbohydrates whenever possible, especially added sugar. Any time I drink juice, I drink less than a half of a glass of juice, with the rest (greater than 60 percent) water (plus ice). My one weakness is too much dark chocolate. However, I have been able to cut this down significantly over the last several years, and instead, I add dark cocoa powder packets (a total of ~500 mg of cocoa flavonols) each day to my drinks. I always choose lean meats, and avoid fried and fatty foods. I drink only skim milk, and choose non-fat or low-fat dairy options when possible. I drink coffee in moderation, eat green leafy vegetables and fruits as often as I can, and fish at least twice per week.

I know first-hand that maintaining a brain-healthy diet can be challenging! As an example, I was recently forced to eat dinner on a short flight from New York to Miami. It was 9 p.m., I was hungry, and my food choices were limited. After takeoff I asked the flight attendant what food they had available for purchase, and she replied, "We have a jumbo-sized cookie, potato chips, or cheese and crackers." Starving, and justifying my expenditure on "market research" purposes for this chapter, I decided to buy all three.

Before deciding which of these would be my dinner for the evening, I read the nutrition labels, as I have become accustomed to over the last several years. Let's start with the cookie: 150 calories; 6 grams fat (3 g saturated, 0 g trans fat); 23 g carbohydrates (0 g dietary fiber, 13 g sugar); 2 g protein. At first glance, the cookie was not as "bad" for me as I had expected. I then double-checked the label and noticed that one cookie actually consisted of three servings! This means I would have needed to triple the amounts above were I to eat the whole thing. At that point I decided to gift the cookie to my friend, Ron, in the seat next to me who ate the cookie and then proceeded to fall asleep and started drooling on my shoulder within minutes (blood sugar crash!).

With my options for dinner dwindling, I reviewed the next option on the menu: the cheese and crackers. This plastic-wrapped tray consisted of four butter crackers (.5 oz, but no nutrition facts), one piece of pasteurized processed cheddar cheese (.75 oz, also no nutrition facts), a box of raisins (90 calories; 0 g fat; 22 g carbohydrates [2 g dietary fiber, 20 g sugar]; 1g protein); and a small bag of mixed nuts (170 calories, 15 g fat (2 g saturated, 0 g trans fat); 6 g carbohydrates [2 g dietary fiber, 1 g, sugar]; 5 g protein).

NOTE: These packaged options illustrate one potential challenge to brain-healthy eating. Many of the foods we eat do not come with nutrition information. There are a number of books and computer programs that provide this information. However, with a little experience, one can "guesstimate" the nutritional contents of foods to a fair degree of accuracy.

The third and final option was the potato chips. This time I noticed the "fine print" staring at me from the top of the nutrition facts label. In this 6-oz container, we have 6 servings (1 oz each) with each serving consisting of 150 calories; 9 g fat (1.5 g satu-

rated, 0 g trans fat); 16 g carbohydrate (1 g dietary fiber, 1g sugars); 1 g protein.

I didn't have to do any math to realize that the options presented to me were suboptimal. When I was younger, I would have started with the cookie, then continued with half (about 3 oz) of the potato chips, and maybe finished with my "dessert" of one piece of cheese and a few of the butter crackers. However, having a family history of AD, I knew I had to put some thought into my food selection. The bag of nuts was an easy first choice. Though they are relatively high in fat, it is mostly unsaturated (good) fat and they provide a fair amount of protein. Next, I moved on to the box of raisins (high in antioxidants). It was at this point, still unsatisfied, I remembered that I had done some simple planning to help me in this scenario. I had saved a "protein bar" in my laptop bag just in case of an event like this. (I had forgotten that I had begun to carry low-glycemic protein bars in all of my travel bags for this very reason). For my beverage, I first had a full glass of water, and then a third of a glass of cranberry juice, mixed with one-third water, and the rest with ice; another easy trick that significantly reduces the carbs in my beverage.

Many clinicians and researchers believe that adopting a Mediterranean-style diet may be helpful toward delaying the onset of AD. Fruits and vegetables, lean protein (fish, chicken, turkey), low-fat foods (especially low in saturated fats), nuts, and seeds are a part of this type of diet. Some advocate for minimizing consumption of red meat (no more than once or twice per week) and also minimizing the amount of processed foods in the diet. When eating dairy products, consider low-fat (or better yet, non-fat) options when possible. In addition, another good general rule of thumb is to choose foods with fewer ingredients listed on the label rather than a long laundry list of unpronounceable additives.

DEFINITION: Mediterranean Diet

This type of type includes plentiful amounts of plant-derived foods and fresh fruit (primary source of carbohydrates), olive oil (primary source of fat), fish and lean poultry (primary source of protein, in low to moderate amounts), red meat (in low amounts), low-fat yogurt and milk (in moderate amounts), and wine (in low to moderate amounts). Regular physical activity is also a part of this diet, which is representative of cultural patterns of eating in countries like Italy, Greece, Spain, and Morocco.

We have talked about the importance of good (unsaturated) fat versus bad (saturated and trans) fat. It is important to learn the difference and make a habit of reading nutrition labels. In fact, it is important to read the Nutrition Facts information and ingredient list on foods when available. Reading labels will help keep track of exactly what is put into the body, which in turn has an effect on brain health.

Eating fish that are high in DHA/EPA is also advisable. There are several specific types of fish, including mackerel, lake trout, herring, sardines, albacore tuna, and wild salmon that are high in these two kinds of omega-3 fatty acids. Tofu and other forms of soybeans may be helpful, as well as canola, walnut, and their oils. Dr. Isaacson advocates for his patients to eat fish in moderation, roughly twice a week, to ensure a good supply of DHA and EPA while mitigating the potential for increasing mercury in the diet. The types of fish that are chosen are also important (wild-caught typically contains higher level of omega-3s as compared to farm-raised).

As discussed in Chapter 12, antioxidants in the diet are essential. Blueberries and strawberries seem to have the strongest evidence of benefits, but several other types of berries are also key (e.g., raspberries, cranberries, acai, cherries, blackberries, and elderberries). We suggest at least one serving per day (while we do not know the exact amount for optimal brain function, the serving size we recommend to our patients is a half cup). As discussed earlier, many vegetables may be quite helpful to protect the brain (e.g., carrots, broccoli, beets, spinach, kale, cabbage, Brussels sprouts, artichokes, collard, and other dark leafy greens). Other popular high-antioxidant foods include dark chocolate (in moderation!), and teas (green and black, but remember no caffeine after lunchtime!).

The effect of alcohol consumption on AD prevention is currently unclear. One serving (in women) or one to two servings (in men) per day may be reasonable. A recent article by Neafsey and Collins concluded that this amount may reduce the risk of dementia and cognitive decline (*Neuropsychiatric Disease and Treatment*, 2011), although further studies are warranted. We advise against consumption of more than two servings per day, as this may lead to significant health consequences. When it comes to treatment, further studies are warranted to determine the effects of alcohol, and this topic should be discussed with the treating physician. In the United States, a "standard" drink contains about 0.6 fluid ounces or 14 grams of "pure" alcohol. Typical servings of alcohol are as follows: 12 oz beer = 8–9 oz malt liquor = 5 oz wine = 3–4 oz fortified wine (e.g., sherry or port) = 2–3 oz cordial liquor (e.g., crème de menthe) = 1.5 oz brandy = 1.5 oz hard liquor (i.e., a shot).

To summarize, we suggest focusing on these general categories of diet and nutrition. When making such dietary changes, it is helpful to keep a diet journal and/or meal log on paper (see Appendix F) or use the AD-NTS as described earlier (visit www.AlzheimersDiet.com for more information). It is also advisable to have laboratory studies (blood work) done before making changes to the diet, as well as several weeks or months afterwards. Again, any and all changes should be under the guidance and strict supervision of a physician and dietician.

TOP-TEN ALZHEIMER'S DIET AND NUTRITION RECOMMENDATIONS

1. Include the following suggested breakdown of macro-nutrients (modified from Craft study):

   - Fat: 25% (less than 7% saturated)

   - Carbohydrates: 30–45% (low-glycemic index)

   - Protein: 25–35%

2. Minimize carbohydrates with a high-glycemic index—especially added simple sugars, high fructose corn syrup, and corn syrup in general. It is unclear what the exact target number of total carbs should be per day, but some

suggest less than 130 grams/day (low-carb diet). Others suggest significantly less, even less than half that amount, for a very low-carbohydrate (ketogenic) diet; however, this is not recommended in our diet plan.

Decrease dietary carbs slowly over weeks and with supervision and approval by a physician (see plan below). Some experts may feel that a very low carbohydrate diet could confer additional benefit over the low carbohydrate diet included in the 9-Week Diet Plan. While this may be true, the potential risk associated with a very low carbohydrate diet prevents us (and most physicians) from making this recommendation to our patients. As mentioned, individuals with specific conditions (e.g., diabetes) must avoid ketogenic diets, as severe health consequences may occur.

3. Try a Mediterranean-style diet, including fruits and vegetables, lean protein (fish, chicken, turkey), low-fat items, nuts, and seeds. Avoid excessive red meat intake as well as processed foods.

4. "Good" fat (unsaturated) versus "bad" fat (saturated and trans fats)—Learn the difference; avoid trans fats, and eat saturated fats in moderation.

5. Omega-3 fatty acids (DHA and EPA) from dietary sources (like fish), as well as additional intake via supplements.

6. Antioxidants. Foods like berries, kale, mushrooms, onions, beans, seeds, sardines, herring, trout, and Alaskan wild salmon demonstrate the variety of foods rich in these brain-boosting components.

7. Vitamins—Ensure adequate intake of folic acid, B6, B12, and vitamin D (via adequate nutrition, and supplement as needed in pill or liquid form).

8. In general, choose foods with as few ingredients listed on the label as possible; the fewer, the better!

9. Select low-fat dairy products (or non-fat) when possible over full-fat products.

10. Coffee (caffeinated): 1–3 cups earlier in the day may be beneficial over time (avoid caffeine after lunchtime to minimize interference with sleep patterns).

Regarding recommendation 2 above, when making dietary suggestions to patients in his clinical practice, Dr. Isaacson suggests the following step-wise approach—the 9-Week Diet Plan—toward dietary enhancement. To avoid potential negative health consequences of dietary modifications such as those discussed in the plan below, supervision by a treating physician is essential. A patient's medical history needs to be considered before any recommendations are followed. As mentioned previously, people with diabetes who are predisposed to ketoacidosis should not follow the 9-Week Diet Plan. Other potential side effects that have been reported from low-carbohydrate diets include constipation or diarrhea, headaches, and muscle weakness. Again, **this plan should only be followed under the supervision of the treating physician.**

PART TWO—THE 9-WEEK DIET PLAN

Changing one's diet is an investment in brain health, which requires some time and effort, particularly in the beginning. Once these things become habit, the time and effort required will be reduced to very little. Our job is to help educate patients and their family members on how to get there, but each person must be prepared to devote the effort required for success.

In the first few weeks, there will be some large tasks to complete (e.g., revamping the home food environment) and some documentation to complete (e.g., food records twice a week in Weeks 1, 4, and 8; carbohydrate tracking daily). Even when there are no daily tasks, we strongly suggest looking at weekly progress and getting into the habit of doing something small but intentional to improve diet *each day*. Again, this is only during the adjustment period of the first several weeks. After this, brain-healthy eating will become second nature. However, this only occurs with continuity in the beginning, meaning that it is essential to stay consistent and invest the effort at the start.

That said, we strongly recommend utilizing the resources provided with The Alzheimer's Diet, including the log sheets in Appendix F and the AD-NTS available at www .AlzheimersDiet.com to record vital dietary information.

Each week, we present guidelines for planning and preparation, eating, and exercise. The checkboxes next to each of these items are provided so they can actually be checked off in paperback versions.

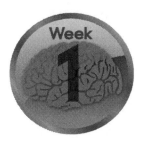

Here is some good news when beginning the Alzheimer's Diet: we can almost guarantee success in the first week! In fact, *we recommend not making any changes to the diet in the first week*. However, there is plenty to be done in preparation for adopting a brain-healthy diet in subsequent weeks. Check off each item as it is completed.

WEEK 1 PLANNING AND PREPARATION

❑ Day 1 (and each first day of the week thereafter): Read through task list below that should be completed in Week 1. This will help in terms of planning for the week, as some items may be done at the same time as other items, and some items (e.g., carbohydrate intake) require daily updates.

❑ Read nutrition labels and ingredient lists on EVERY food item that is eaten. See Chapter 19 for tips on what to look for on nutrition labels.

❑ Record carbohydrates each day of the week on the diet journal log sheets (Appendix F) or electronically in the AD-NTS Carbohydrate Tracker found at www .AlzheimersDiet.com.

❏ Complete two days of food records (one weekday and one weekend day). **Record everything you eat and drink** on those days, including ingredients, additions, and condiments. Although it is not necessary to record nutritional information, pay particular attention to the important nutritional information of the items you list (e.g., glycemic index and load of carbohydrates, types of protein, saturated fat, unsaturated fat) prior to making dietary changes. A variety of websites and handbooks provide estimates of the macronutrient content of different foods (e.g., http://ndb.nal.usda.gov/ or http://www.nal.usda.gov/fnic/foodcomp/Data/HG72/hg72_2002.pdf or http://nutritiondata.self.com/). Food record information can be recorded either on plain notebook paper (don't lose it!) or electronically via the AD-NTS found at www.AlzheimersDiet.com. Examples of good and bad food records are also available on the AD-NTS.

❏ Identify three favorite brain-*unhealthy* snacks and three favorite brain-*unhealthy* meals. Record this information in the back of the book (Appendix F) or on the AD-NTS website (www.AlzheimersDiet.com). This will give a record of the largest dietary "offenders," which we will replace or change in upcoming weeks.

❏ Identify any challenges to revamping the home food environment. Record this information in the back of the book (Appendix F) or on the AD-NTS website (www.AlzheimersDiet.com).

❏ Identify two potential solutions to each challenge to revamping the home food environment. Record this information in the back of the book (Appendix F) or on the AD-NTS website (www.AlzheimersDiet.com).

❏ Go food shopping at different health food stores and explore the healthy and natural food aisle in the grocery store. Purchase three new brain-healthy snacks. Read nutrition labels to identify brain-healthy snacks (i.e., low glycemic, low saturated fat, antioxidant rich). See chapter 19 for tips on food shopping and reading nutrition labels.

❏ Inform family about changes that will be made to accommodate a brain-healthy diet. This serves three purposes: 1) Household members will expect changes in the home food environment and know why; 2) Having advocates and allies through this process makes it easier and more fun; and 3) Announcing these behavioral changes makes an individual more accountable to others and, in turn, more likely to stick with the changes.

❏ Identify and write down one exercise that could be done for at least 20 minutes three times per week. Note: all exercise should be approved by the treating physician and appropriate to the individual's level of fitness. Remember three important things: 1) Exercise does not need to be overly strenuous or require sweat or a gym to be effective; 2) The benefits of exercise are additive, so 5 minutes done four times in a day is the same as 20 minutes in one sitting (this could as simple as taking the stairs instead of the elevator or walking around the block); and 3) Find something enjoyable (e.g., sports activities). The more enjoyable the exercise, the more likely it is to be sustained long term. Record this information in the back of the book (Appendix F) or on the AD-NTS website (www.The Alzheimers Diet.com).

❏ At the end of the week, review the carbohydrate logs and food records for the week. Our patients put a lot of effort into these logs, and they should put them to use! These logs are a wealth of information and will help to identify where dietary changes are necessary.

WEEK 1 EATING

❏ Do not make any dietary changes yet.

WEEK 1 EXERCISE

❏ Do not make any changes to exercise yet.

Week 1 will help people become mindful of what they are eating, identify where attention needs to be focused, become accustomed to reading nutrition labels at the supermarket and prepare for changes in Week 2. Future weeks will build on this preparatory work, so be sure to complete each step before advancing. If, for any reason, an individual cannot complete these steps in one week, it is fine to complete these in two weeks. It is more important that individuals complete each step and follow this process at a pace that works for them. Remember, these changes are meant to be for the rest of one's life!

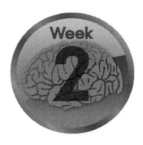

Week 2 will be the largest transition week. We will focus on changing the home food environment and trying some new brain-healthy foods.

WEEK 2 PLANNING AND PREPARATION

❏ Day 1: Read through the task list below of things to complete in Week 2.

❏ Read nutrition labels on EVERY food item that is eaten.

❏ No food records this week, but **it is essential to keep track of total grams of carbohydrates**. Record carbohydrates each day of the week on the diet journal log sheets (Appendix F) or electronically in the AD-NTS Carbohydrate Tracker found at www.AlzheimersDiet.com.

❏ Revamp the home food environment. As discussed, the food environment has the single largest effect on what a person eats. We want to limit the availability of brain-unhealthy foods and make brain-healthy foods readily available. Therefore, this is will involve two stages: 1) Ridding the household of brain unhealthy items; and 2) Stocking the household with brain-healthy items. Do this in the beginning of the week, as it will be essential for the week's diet plan.

• **Stage I:** Rid the household of brain-unhealthy items. Although nobody likes to waste food, we need to get brain-unhealthy items out of the home. Donate or throw away full-fat dairy products (milk, mayonnaise, canola oil, full-fat salad dressings, etc.). Make a list of the full-fat items discarded so they can be replaced with low or no fat versions in Stage II. Remember, getting rid of items and ingredients that will not be noticed should be easy. When it comes to favorite brain-unhealthy snacks, a balance is needed; we do not want people to be miserable because they are missing a favorite food. By the same token, the benefit of the diet will reflect the level of effort put into it. If individuals have items on their list that are serious brain offenders, we do not recommend telling them that they can never consume these things again, but we *strongly* recommend not keeping these items in the household.

• **Stage II:** Stock the household with brain-healthy items. This will be the largest single investment in terms of cost. We suggest shopping at different grocery and health food stores to get a feel for which places carry preferred items. Take the list of discarded items and replace as many as possible with low- or non-fat versions. Also take the Week 1 list of favorite brain-unhealthy meals and replace as many of the ingredients with brain-healthy options as possible (e.g., cooking spray instead of oil, low- or no-fat cheese, lean instead of high-fat meat products, vegetables instead of potatoes, etc.) Purchase at least one piece of fresh fish to eat this week. Purchase three new brain-healthy snacks (so there will be six in the household, including the three purchased in Week 1). Finally, make sure to purchase at least one new antioxidant-rich food or dietary supplement (such as dark cocoa powder).

❏ *Optional: Enter Week 1 food record information into the nutrition analysis tool at www.fitday.com or http://www.myfood record.com/mainnat.html. This will provide a snapshot of dietary composition before beginning the diet, which can be printed and referred to again later.*

WEEK 2 EATING

❏ Try three of the six new brain-healthy snacks this week.

❏ Record which new brain-healthy snacks were tried with an evaluation of each (scale of one to ten, with ten being the best and one being the worst). Record this information in the back of the book (Appendix F) or on the AD-NTS website (www.AlzheimersDiet.com).

❏ Replace one of the favorite *meals* identified in Week 1 with brain-healthy ingredients, making it a brain-healthy meal.

❏ Once approved by (and under close supervision of) a physician, reduce carbohydrate intake to a goal of 130–150 grams of carbohydrates per day.

❏ Minimize high-glycemic carbohydrates (see http://www .mendosa.com/gilists.htm for a list of the glycemic index and glycemic load of most foods).

❏ Begin efforts to follow the general breakdown of macronutrients (protein, fat, and carbohydrates) per day as described in the first part of this chapter and increase lean meats and low-fat options, while decreasing simple and added sugars.

❑ Eat fish at least twice this week.

❑ Have at least one serving of fruit or vegetable each day.

WEEK 2 EXERCISE

❑ Try the exercise identified in Week 1 at least once this week. This means 20 minutes of exercise throughout the week (that should be doable for everyone!). Note: The recommendation to start slow is directed toward relatively sedentary individuals; however, more active individuals may want to do more. As long as it is approved by the treating physician, more exercise is generally better.

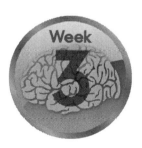

Now that the home food environment is prepared and some minor adjustments in actual diet have been made, we should be ready for more advanced dietary changes in Week 3.

WEEK 3 PLANNING AND PREPARATION

❏ Read through task list below of things to complete in Week 3.

❏ Read nutrition labels on EVERY food item that is eaten.

❏ No food records this week, but **it is essential to keep track of total grams of carbohydrates**. Record carbohydrates each day of the week on the diet journal log sheets (Appendix F) or electronically in the AD-NTS Carbohydrate Tracker found at www.AlzheimersDiet.com.

❏ Identify and write down the top three brain-healthy snacks. Record this information in the back of the book (Appendix F) or on the AD-NTS website (www .AlzheimersDiet.com).

❏ Purchase ingredients for a new brain-healthy meal (if the ingredients are not already in the home). Some brain-healthy meal suggestions are included in Appendices D and E, but creating one's own meals from brain-healthy ingredients is important. Remember, experimenting with and finding several satisfying go-to brain-healthy meals is essential to making one's brain and belly happy at the same time. While at the food store, purchase more of the top-three brain-healthy snacks identified above. Fill the home with these! Remember, we generally reach for what is readily available, so filling the home with brain-healthy snacks will drastically increase consumption of those foods.

❏ Identify at least two challenges to brain-healthy eating in the home. Record this information in the back of the book (Appendix F) or on the AD-NTS website (www .AlzheimersDiet.com).

❏ Identify and write down two potential solutions to each challenge. Record this information in the back of the book (Appendix F) or on the AD-NTS website (www .AlzheimersDiet.com).

❏ Identify one new exercise that could be done for at least 20 minutes three times per week. Record this information in the back of the book (Appendix F) or electronically via the AD-NTS found at www.AlzheimersDiet.com. The goal is to have some choice and to try different varieties until individuals find exercises they truly enjoy doing.

WEEK 3 EATING

❏ Try the other three new brain-healthy snacks this week.

❏ Record which new brain-healthy snacks were tried with an evaluation of each (scale of one to ten, with ten being the best and one being the worst). Record this information in the back of the book (Appendix F) or electronically via the AD-NTS found at www.AlzheimersDiet.com.

❏ Aim for a goal of 110–130 grams of carbohydrates per day.

❏ Minimize high-glycemic carbohydrates (see http://www .mendosa.com/gilists.htm).

❏ Follow the general breakdown of macronutrients (protein, fat, and carbohydrates) per day as described in the first part of this chapter.

❏ Continue a step-wise increase in lean meats and low-fat options, while decreasing simple and added sugars.

❏ Eat fish at least twice this week. Experiment with different recipes (just not fried). Although we can provide suggestions, it is vital that each person create their own for two reasons: 1) Each individual is different and only he or she knows what flavors he or she prefers, and 2) Creating one's own brain-healthy recipes is a tremendous and necessary learning tool for dietary changes to be carried out through the rest of one's life.

❏ Continue to increase foods rich in antioxidants, and increase fruits and vegetables.

❏ Replace one other of the favorite *meals* identified in Week 1 with brain-healthy ingredients, making it a brain-healthy meal.

❏ Have at least one serving of fruit or vegetable each day.

WEEK 3 EXERCISE

❏ In addition to the time spent walking around food stores (which is exercise), perform the exercise identified in Week 1 at least once this week. That means 20 minutes of exercise throughout the week.

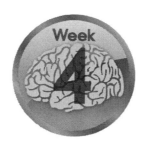

Now that the home food environment is brain-healthy, we will focus on executing what has been learned and prepared for in prior weeks, as well as preparing for eating outside of the home.

WEEK 4 PLANNING AND PREPARATION

❑ Read through the task list of things to complete in Week 4.

❑ Read nutrition labels on EVERY food item that is eaten.

❑ Record carbohydrates each day of the week on the diet journal log sheets (Appendix F) or electronically in the AD-NTS Carbohydrate Tracker found at www .Alzheimers Diet.com.

❑ Complete two days of food records this week (one weekday and one weekend day). At nearly the halfway point through the 9-Week Plant transition, this will provide information on the changes made so far and identify which areas require the most effort going forward. Record this information on regular notebook paper or electronically in the AD-NTS found at www.AlzheimersDiet.com.

❑ Examine food records closely. After working to do them,

put them to work for you! Identify areas that can be optimized to become more brain-healthy.

❏ Record carbohydrates each day of the week on the diet journal log sheets (Appendix F) or electronically in the AD-NTS Carbohydrate Tracker found at www .AlzheimersDiet.com.

❏ Plan for eating outside of the home. Most people eat multiple meals outside the home each week. Identify and record at least two brain-healthy meals (aside from a meal replacement) that could be consumed for breakfast, lunch, and dinner outside the home (even if you take something from home, which we encourage). Also, identify and record at least two brain-healthy meals that could be ordered at the most frequented restaurant(s) for breakfast, lunch, and dinner. Record this information in the back of the book (Appendix F) or electronically via the AD-NTS found at www.AlzheimersDiet.com.

WEEK 4 EATING

❏ Eat 110–130 grams of carbohydrates per day.

❏ Minimize high-glycemic carbohydrates (see http://www .mendosa.com/gilists.htm).

❏ Follow the breakdown of macronutrients (protein, fat, and carbohydrates) per day as described in the first part of this chapter.

❏ Continue a step-wise increase in lean meats and low-fat options, while decreasing simple and added sugars.

❏ Eat fish at least twice this week.

❏ Continue to increase foods rich in antioxidants, and increase fruits and vegetables.

❏ Have at least one serving of fruit or vegetable each day, especially brain-healthy berries like blueberries and strawberries once or twice per week.

❏ Replace the last of the favorite *meals* identified in Week 1 with brain-healthy ingredients, making it a brain-healthy meal.

WEEK 4 EXERCISE

❏ Perform the exercise identified in Week 1 at least once this week for 20 minutes and try the new exercise identified in Week 3 for 20 minutes at least once this week. That means at least 40 minutes of exercise throughout the week, as tolerated and as approved by the treating physician.

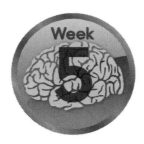

At a little over the halfway point of the diet transition period, significant changes have been made to the home food environment, the diet (both in and out of the home), and exercise habits. The remaining weeks will be spent tightening and tweaking the diet so it suits the needs of each individual. At this point, feeling comfortable experimenting with new foods and being able to "guestimate" nutritional content of foods before looking at labels should be the norm. Guesstimating can be fun, so have fun with it, but always confirm the amounts.

WEEK 5 PLANNING AND PREPARATION

❏ Read through the task list of things to complete in Week 5.

❏ Read nutrition labels on EVERY food item that is eaten, but first try to **guess the important nutrient contents before reading the label.**

❏ No food records this week, but **it is essential to keep track of total grams of carbohydrates.** Record carbohydrates each day of the week on the diet journal log sheets (Appendix F) or electronically in the AD-NTS Carbohydrate Tracker found at www.AlzheimersDiet.com.

❏ Identify and write down at least two challenges to brain-healthy eating outside the home.

❏ Identify and write down two potential solutions to each challenge.

❏ Identify and write down one new exercise that could be done for at least 20 minutes three times per week. Although individuals may already have favorite exercises established, it is important to think about new exercises in order to recognize additional opportunities to improve health and how these may fit into one's daily routine. Record this information in the back of the book (Appendix F) or electronically via the AD-NTS found at www.AlzheimersDiet.com.

❏ *Optional: Enter Week 4 food record information into the nutrition analysis tool at www.fitday.com or http://www.myfood record.com/mainnat.html. This will provide a snapshot of dietary composition halfway through The 9-Week Diet Plan adoption period. This can be printed and compared to Week 1's information.*

WEEK 5 EATING

❏ Try to decrease carbohydrates to 90–110 grams per day.

❏ Minimize high-glycemic carbohydrates (see http://www.mendosa.com/gilists.htm).

❏ Eat fish at least twice this week.

❑ Continue a step-wise increase in lean meats and low-fat options, while decreasing simple and added sugars.

❑ Continue to increase foods rich in antioxidants.

❑ Increase fruit and vegetable intake to at least two servings each day. For example, this could be an apple as a snack or with lunch and a vegetable with dinner. A large spinach salad for lunch would also count as two servings.

WEEK 5 EXERCISE

❑ Perform any combination of the exercises identified in Week 1 and Week 3 at least twice this week for 20 minutes. That means at least 40 minutes of exercise throughout the week.

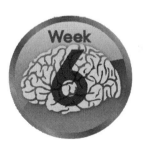

Week 6 provides the opportunity to adjust to the changes made in Week 5. Make sure to note any challenges that arise and problem-solve as soon as possible. Although unanticipated, any adverse dietary or gastrointestinal (digestive system) effects should be reported to the treating physician immediately.

Remaining weeks will focus on decreasing carbohydrates further, separated in two-week increments in order to allow individuals to adjust to these changes before making further reductions in carbohydrate intake.

WEEK 6 PLANNING AND PREPARATION

❏ Read through the task list of things to complete in Week 6.

❏ Read nutrition labels on EVERY food item that is eaten but guess the important nutrient contents before reading the label.

❏ No food records this week, but **it is essential to keep track of total grams of carbohydrates**. Record carbohydrates each day of the week on the diet journal log sheets (Appendix F) or electronically in the AD-NTS Carbohydrate Tracker found at www.AlzheimersDiet.com.

❏ Identify and write down one *new* brain-healthy meal. It is essential to experiment with new ingredients and meals to identify those that are satisfying to the belly as well as the brain. Record this information in the back of the book (Appendix F) or electronically via the AD-NTS found at www.AlzheimersDiet.com.

WEEK 6 EATING

❏ Eat 90–110 grams of carbohydrates per day.

❏ Minimize high-glycemic carbohydrates (see http://www .mendosa.com/gilists.htm).

❑ Eat fish at least twice this week.

❑ Have at least two servings of fruit or vegetables each day.

WEEK 6 EXERCISE

❑ Perform any combination of the exercises identified in Week 1 and Week 3 at least twice this week for 20 minutes. In addition, try the new exercise identified in Week 5 for 20 minutes at least once this week. That means at least 60 minutes of exercise throughout the week.

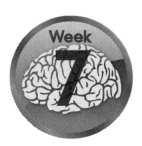

Week 7 focuses on a further reduction in carbohydrate intake.

WEEK 7 PLANNING AND PREPARATION

❑ Read through the task list of things to complete in Week 7.

❑ Read nutrition labels on EVERY food item that is eaten but guess the important nutrient contents before reading the label.

❑ No food records this week, but **it is essential to keep track of total grams of carbohydrates**. Record carbohydrates each day of the week on the diet journal log sheets (Appendix F) or electronically in the AD-NTS Carbohydrate Tracker found at www.AlzheimersDiet.com.

WEEK 7 EATING

❏ Try to decrease carbohydrates to 80–100 grams per day. Note: if any symptoms of ketoacidosis occur, increase the amount of carbohydrates in the diet and speak with the primary-care doctor or treating physician immediately. If symptoms are moderate or severe, go to the emergency room or see the primary care doctor or supervising physician immediately. Early signs of ketoacidosis include increasing fatigue, tired and sleepy, weakness, increased thirst, frequent urination, dry skin and tongue, leg cramps, fruity odor to the breath, upset stomach, nausea. Later signs of ketoacidosis include vomiting, shortness of breath, and increased breathing rate or pulse.

❏ Minimize high-glycemic carbohydrates (see http://www .mendosa.com/gilists.htm).

❏ Try the new brain-healthy meal identified in Week 6.

❏ Eat fish at least twice this week.

❏ Have at least two servings of fruit or vegetables each day.

WEEK 7 EXERCISE

❏ Perform any combination of the exercises identified for at least 20 minutes three times (for a total of at least 60 minutes) this week.

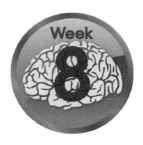

Week 8 provides additional time to adjust to the further reduction in carbohydrate intake recommended in Week 7. There is only one more week left in The 9-Week Diet Plan adoption period!

WEEK 8 PLANNING AND PREPARATION

❏ Read through the task list of things to complete in Week 8.

❏ Read nutrition labels on EVERY food item that is eaten but guess the important nutrient contents before reading the label.

❏ Record carbohydrates each day of the week on the diet journal log sheets (Appendix F) or electronically in the AD-NTS Carbohydrate Tracker found at www .AlzheimersDiet.com.

❏ Complete two entries of food records (one weekday and one weekend day, like in Weeks 1 and 4). At nearly the end of the 9-week diet transition, this will help provide information on the changes made thus far and identify any areas that require further effort going forward. Record on regular notebook paper or electronically in the AD-NTS found at www.AlzheimersDiet.com.

❏ Rate the three exercises tried so far according to enjoyment and sustainability. Record on regular notebook paper or electronically via the AD-NTS found at www.AlzheimersDiet.com.

WEEK 8 EATING

❏ Eat 75–95 grams of carbohydrates per day

❏ Minimize high-glycemic carbohydrates (see http://www .mendosa.com/gilists.htm).

❏ Eat fish at least twice this week.

❏ Have at least two servings of fruit or vegetables each day.

WEEK 8 EXERCISE

❏ Perform the preferred exercises for at least 20 minutes three times (for a total of at least 60 minutes) this week.

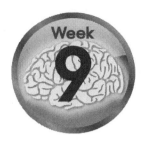

In the last week of the 9-Week Diet Plan, we recommend a final incremental decrease in carbohydrate intake. It is important to note that we are not advocating for a very low-carbohydrate or "ketogenic" diet. Although there is some evidence to suggest that this *may* be helpful for people with Alzheimer's disease, a ketogenic diet presents a higher risk of adverse side effects and should be attempted only under advisement and very strict guidance of a physician and registered dietician. **Important: People with diabetes and other medical conditions (or those taking certain medications) should avoid ketogenic diets, as severe health consequences may occur.** Further, ketogenic diets are quite restrictive and difficult to maintain long term. Remember, the goal of the Alzheimer's Diet is to transform dietary habits for the rest of one's life. Although dietary adjustment requires significant effort in the beginning, it should not be a burden after it becomes habit!

WEEK 9 PLANNING AND PREPARATION

❏ Read through the task list of things to complete in Week 9.

❏ Read nutrition labels on EVERY food item that is eaten

but guess the important nutrient contents before reading the label.

❏ No food records this week, but **it is essential to keep track of total grams of carbohydrates.** Record carbohydrates each day of the week on the diet journal log sheets (Appendix F) or electronically in the AD-NTS Carbohydrate Tracker found at www.AlzheimersDiet.com.

❏ List the Top Ten brain-healthy snacks and meals eaten over the 9-week period. Record this information in the back of the book (Appendix F) or electronically via the AD-NTS found at www.AlzheimersDiet.com.

❏ *Optional: Enter Week 8 food record information into the nutrition analysis tool at www.fitday.com or http://www.myfood record.com/mainnat.html. This will provide a snapshot of dietary composition after the majority of brain-healthy eating has been adopted and can be compared to information from Weeks 1 and 4. See progress!*

WEEK 9 EATING

❏ Decrease carbs to 75 grams or less per day, if tolerated. If symptoms of ketoacidosis occur (see symptoms in previous section), increase the amount of carbohydrates and speak with the primary-care doctor or treating physician. If symptoms are moderate or severe, go to the emergency room or see a primary-care or supervising physician immediately.

❏ Minimize high-glycemic carbohydrates (see http://www .mendosa.com/gilists.htm).

❏ Eat fish at least twice this week.

❏ Have at least two servings of fruit or vegetable each day.

WEEK 9 EXERCISE

❏ Perform the preferred exercises for at least 20 minutes three times (for a total of at least 60 minutes) this week.

BEYOND WEEK 9

If you have reached this point, you have dedicated significant effort toward changing your diet and increasing exercise—congratulations! If the steps in the 9-Week Diet Plan are completed in order, brain-healthy eating should now be a habit and almost second nature. Although it is always important to be aware of one's diet, it is no longer be necessary to formally document information. However, we strongly recommend reviewing the strategies described in this book, initially following the 9-Week Diet Plan, and reviewing the information recorded in the back of the book (Appendix F) or electronically in the AD-NTS at www.AlzheimersDiet.com. This is particularly important when the dreaded "diet fatigue" sets in. This is where some people grow tired of their diet and begin to revert back to unhealthy habits. If this occurs, read this book again and focus on changing habits that require the least noticeable sacrifice. Remember, keep the belly happy. Everyone should love their diet!

BEYOND WEEK 9 PLANNING AND PREPARATION

Planning and preparation are not just for making major changes to one's diet but also for maintaining them. Plan and prepare for future challenges to brain-healthy eating such as vacations, holidays, and parties. Also prepare for stressful periods (e.g., moving, work transitions, having extended family visiting), during which following any kind of diet may be more challenging. Think ahead, prepare early, and always carry a brain-healthy meal replacement for emergencies. This way, brain-healthy options are always available.

BEYOND WEEK 9 EATING

Continue the recommendations of the Alzheimer's Diet as tolerated and, particularly, continue to minimize high-glycemic carbohydrates. By this time, everyone should be familiar with the concepts and challenges associated with brain-healthy eating (both in and outside the home) and should have several strategies in place for dealing with those challenges. The home food environment should be stocked with a number of brain-healthy snacks and meal ingredients, and when dining out, strategies for brain-healthy eating should be at the ready. **Perhaps most important: everyone should now be familiar enough with the nutritional breakdown, particularly the carbohydrate content, of the majority of foods they eat.** For unfamiliar foods, important information can be derived from nutrition labels. At this point, everyone should be in the habit of checking the nutritional content of everything they eat!

Remember, eating can and should be both brain healthy and enjoyable! As the old proverb goes, the idea of this book and particularly the tasks in the 9-Week Diet Plan are not intended to feed people, but to teach them how to fish. If someone is feeling unsure whether he or she possess the skills necessary to sustain this diet for life, we recommend reviewing all of the materials completed here or on the AD-NTS site. Looked at collectively, this information provides:

- Detailed nutritional information at the beginning, middle, and end of the 9-Week Diet Plan.

- Strategies for dealing with challenges to acquiring and maintaining a brain-healthy home food environment.

- Strategies for dealing with challenges to brain-healthy eating outside the home.

- A list of favorite brain-healthy snacks and meals.

- A list of enjoyable and practical exercises.

Continue practicing the good habits formed over the past nine weeks: eat fish at least twice per week; have at least two servings of fruits or vegetables each day; and limit carbohydrates, particularly high-glycemic carbohydrates. In addition, continue to experiment with new brain-healthy ingredients and meals. Again, it is vital to keep the belly, as well as the brain, happy if a diet is going to be maintained.

BEYOND WEEK 9 EXERCISE

❏ Continue performing any combination of the exercises

identified. Continue to try new exercises and incorporate them into the daily routine in weeks to come. We recommend at least 20 minutes of exercise at least three times per week *minimum*. This means that, of the 10,080 minutes in a week, at least 60 of them will be spent exercising. Remember, as long as it is approved by the treating physician, the more the better. Finally, make sure it is fun!

DR. ISAACSON:

I have tried to make an honest effort over the last several years to follow the suggestions that I advocate for. There are some days and weeks where I am quite disciplined, and others where I am less adherent. It is important to not let frustration get the best of you and to realize that even subtle dietary changes for a few days per week, or a few weeks per month, may lead to long-term benefits when followed for many years in a row.

CHAPTER 19

Grocery Shopping

Note: Several examples of food choices to consider, and which choices may be better for optimal brain health, can be found in the appendices. There is also a section on food terminology for better understanding the dietary choices that present themselves throughout the day.

As mentioned earlier, we highly recommend refreshing all of the groceries in the home food environment. This means getting rid of all or at least most brain-unhealthy food products and ingredients and replacing

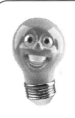

KEY CONCEPT: Don't fill the house with stuff that is bad for one's brain!

them with brain-healthy substitutions. This alone will make a drastic difference in one's diet. **Thus, one trip to the supermarket could literally change your life and improve your memory.**

READING FOOD LABELS

Nutrition labels can be confusing for many people. In fact, a number of studies have shown that even most college-educated people in the United States cannot accurately interpret the information provided. Hopefully, the following tips will help you decipher the "code." The following are the main things to look for on nutrition labels:

- *Number of servings per container.* People typically assume that a container of food (e.g., bottle of soda) contains 1 serving. Many times a container contains two or more servings. Therefore, if the entire container is consumed, the rest of the nutrition facts must be multiplied by the number of servings in that container. In the example above, the container contains about 4 servings and 540 (135 x 4) calories.

NUTRITION FACTS		
Serving Size 8 fl oz (240ml)		
Servings Per Container About 4		
Amount Per Serving		
Calories 135		Calories from Fat 0
		% Daily Value*
Total Fat	0g	0%
Saturated Fat	0g	0%
Trans Fat	0g	
Cholesterol	0mg	0%
Sodium	25mg	1%
Total Carbohydrate	34g	11%
Dietary Fiber	0mg	0%
Sugars	28g	
Protein	0g	
Vitamin A 2%		Vitamin C 35%
Calcium 10%		Iron 6%

* Percent Daily Values Are Based On A 2000 Calorie Diet. Your daily values may be higher or lower depending on your calorie needs:

		2,000	2,500
Total Fat	Less than	65g	80g
Sat Fat	Less than	20g	25g
Cholesterol	Less than	300mg	300mg
Sodium	Less than	2,400mg	2,400mg
Total Carbohydrate		300g	375g
Dietary Fiber		25g	30g

- *Fat, particularly saturated and trans fat.* As we have discussed, steer clear of trans fat. Strive to keep saturated fat to less than 7 percent of total daily calories. Unfortunately, this is not directly listed on food labels, so it must be estimated. The average normal weight (BMI 18.5–24.9) woman consumes approximately 2,000 calories per day, and should consume less than 15 grams of saturated fat per day. The average normal weight (BMI 18.5–24.9) man consumes approximately 2500 calories per day, and should consume less than 19 grams of saturated fat per day.

- **Carbohydrates.** Nutrition labels list the total carbohydrate content in grams (see 9-Week Diet Plan for specific recommendations) but do not provide any information as to whether they are good or bad carbs. See Chapters 2, 4, and 9 for this information.

- **Fiber.** Generally speaking, more is better when it comes to dietary fiber.

- **Sugar.** Remember, sugar is considered a simple (bad) carbohydrate so less sugar is better in terms of carbohydrate content.

- **Protein.** Nutrition labels list the total protein content in grams but do not provide any information on the quality of the protein. See Chapter 11 for this information. In general, food items that have a total calorie to gram of protein ratio of 10 : 1 are considered high protein. For example, a chicken breast sandwich may have 400 calories and 40 grams of protein (10 : 1 calorie to gram protein ratio).

INGREDIENTS

The more brain-healthy ingredients, the more brain-healthy the meal! We highly recommend replacing all unhealthy ingredients (fatty dressings and condiments, such as mayonnaise) with brain-healthy ingredients. As we have discussed, these substitutions may include fat-free versions of cream, cheese, mayonnaise and salad dressings, less unhealthy butter substitutes such as I Can't Believe It's Not Butter, cooking spray instead of oil, lean instead of fatty beef, fish instead of pork, vegetables instead of potatoes, and rye or whole grain instead of white bread.

SNACKS

All else being equal, the more a person eats of one thing, the less he or she eats of another. That means that even if the only change an individual made was to purchase additional household snacks that were brain healthy, they would likely not only eat more brain-healthy snacks but also eat fewer brain-unhealthy snacks. We encourage reducing temptation even further by purchasing only or mostly brain-healthy snacks. Brain-healthy snacks or "starters," including clear soups and salads, may also help prevent overeating less healthy main courses. For these reasons, we encourage loading up on brain-healthy snacks to have around the home at all times.

BEVERAGES

Beverages are frequently ignored in dietary planning, but can have a very large impact on the overall brain health of one's diet.

Beverages can be an unsuspected source of poor carbohydrates (sugar) that will cause the dramatic spike in blood sugar and subsequent crash we have been trying to teach you to avoid. For example, there are 65 g of sugar in a typical 20 oz bottle of cola. That's about 15 teaspoons of sugar!

A common complaint when attempting to switch to diet soda is palatability. There is no denying the taste difference between diet and non-diet cola but again the question is, "Is it worth it?" **For one's brain, yes.**

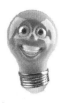

KEY CONCEPT: Do not buy sugared beverages! This includes beverages sweetened by high fructose corn syrup (same thing as sugar).

Although juice certainly provides more nutrition than do sodas, beware some juices contain nearly the same amount of carbohydrate/glucose. Different juices (even 100 percent juice) have very different glycemic profiles. For example most apple juices have a glycemic index in the high 30s, while most orange juices have a glycemic index in the mid 50s. Also, beware of products labeled "juice beverage," "juice cocktail," and "juice drink." These are not juice! Most contain a little (e.g., 15 percent) juice and the rest is sugar or high fructose corn syrup. For example, most fruit juices have a glycemic index between 35 and 55, and a glycemic load between 10 and 15. Compare that to typical cranberry juice cocktail, which has a glycemic index of almost 70 and a glycemic load of 24. Vegetable juices may have an even better glycemic profile than even 100 percent fruit juices, but be wary of added salt and sugar.

Alcohol is another frequently unsuspected offender. Beer and wine vary in their sugar and caloric content but be aware that *all* beers and wines contain some carbohydrates and more calories than most individuals expect. Straight liquor (e.g., vodka, gin, whisky) typically does not provide carbohydrates but still contains a significant number of calories (about 100 per shot) and are typically mixed with sugary beverages that deliver carbohydrates and even more calories. If anything, we recommend red wine in moderation, due to the flavonoid content mentioned earlier.

CHAPTER 20

Restaurant Eating

When it comes to following a brain-healthy diet, restaurant eating can be one of the most challenging aspects. This is partly why we recommend preparing as much food as possible at home. However, some people will still eat out frequently, so they need to take special care to be sure to avoid brain-unhealthy meals. Even seemingly healthy restaurant dishes such as chicken and vegetables may contain large amounts of fat and saturated fat. Chefs are notorious for sautéing in butter and/or oil, rendering what could have been a brain-healthy food into to a brain-bruising food loaded with saturated fat. It's always a good idea to ask how your food is going to be prepared and then request brain-healthy modifications if necessary.

The following are some hidden dangers to watch for:

- Buttered sandwich buns

- "Breaded" or "tempura" items (This typically means the food has been deep-fried.)

- Sautéed foods (This typically means the food has been sautéed in oil.)

- Salad dressing (A salad should be fairly brain healthy, but restaurant dressings are usually high in saturated fats.)

- The addition of butter and/or oil to foods like potatoes, vegetables, rice, couscous, risotto, and other "sticky" foods.

- Food cooked on flattop grills (Food cooked on flattop grills tend to sit in a pool of grease and absorb large amounts of saturated fat.)

- Fruit tarts and other seemingly healthy desserts (Just because it sounds healthy doesn't mean it isn't loaded with sugar. Order a fresh fruit cup with as many berries as possible instead.)

Here are some simple rules of thumb to follow, which should make dining out a little healthier:

- Avoid butter or cream sauces. (Opt for tomato sauce instead.)

- Avoid fried items. (Choose baked or broiled alternatives.)

- Avoid foods typically prepared with oil. (Request no or light oil in the preparation of your food.)

- If you are not sure about what's going into your food or how it is going to be prepared, ask! There's no reason to feel embarrassed about looking out for your health.

- Choose either an appetizer or a dessert. These items typically contain the most saturated fat, so practice moderation and cut one out instead of ordering both. Or request fresh fruit for dessert.

- Pass on the bread before the meal. Bread typically contains empty carbs and a lot of calories. Remember, high-glycemic equals blood sugar spike equals bad for memory!

- Drink diet soda, water, or non-sweetened tea (with an artificial sweetener, if necessary).

- Limit alcohol consumption with the meal; if you have a mixed drink, choose a non-caloric mixer.

The idea is to know how to order before sitting down in the restaurant and being caught off guard. It's not necessary for someone to know *exactly what* they will order, but they should have already made firm decisions about appetizers, desserts, bread, and drinks. Once an individual finds a regimen that works for them for restaurant eating, he or she should stick to it. This does not mean ordering the same things every time, but the more structured the experience, the easier it will be to stay on track with brain-healthy eating.

CHAPTER 21

Parties, Peer Pressure, and Other Challenges

In the United States, following a particular diet is much easier than it used to be. Almost everyone is on some kind of diet these days, and people are becoming more accepting and accommodating when it comes to party food. It is relatively common for someone throwing a party to have at least a few healthy options available. Look for lean protein, particularly from fish or chicken that may be served. Just beware that these things are typically prepared with butter 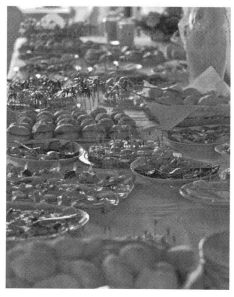 and/or oil. If you can, check with the host or hostess to see what is on the menu. You can even offer to bring a brain-healthy dish. If that is not feasible, it is a good idea to eat prior to the party so that impulsive eating can be avoided. Also, a meal-replacement bar might come in handy while everyone else is snacking on sugary cakes and cookies!

COMMON PARTY MENU ITEMS
TO STAY AWAY FROM:

- Pigs in a blanket

- Anything fried (e.g., chicken fingers)

- Cream- and cheese-based dips (e.g., ranch dressing, vegetable dip, nacho cheese dip)

- Almost anything that came frozen from a bag (e.g., mini quiches, mini egg rolls, spring rolls)

- Pretzels and chips

- Pizza

- Loaded potato skins

- Cookies, cakes, and pies

BRAIN-HEALTHY OPTIONS FREQUENTLY
SEEN AT PARTIES:

- Shrimp cocktail. As long as the shrimp are not fried or prepared in oil, they are an excellent option. Use cocktail sauce sparingly; although it contains relatively little if any saturated fat, the ketchup still contains bad carbohydrates.

- Vegetables. Many parties will feature a vegetable platter. Just be aware that the dip is typically loaded with saturated fat and carbohydrates. If hummus is available, go for that.

- Fruit platter

- Nuts

- Sushi. Although the rice will contain some carbs, sushi is still a relatively good choice if available.

- Wraps. Vegetable and or ham and turkey wraps are fairly good options, particularly if the wraps are whole grain.

- Turkey and/or ham deli sandwiches. Use mustard instead of mayonnaise and consider removing the bread or at least half of the bread (make it an "open face sandwich"), particularly if it is white bread.

- Salsa. Although tortilla chips contain bad carbohydrates and typically some saturated fat, salsa is nearly all chopped vegetables and makes a much better dip or topping than other alternatives such as ranch dressing or cheese dip.

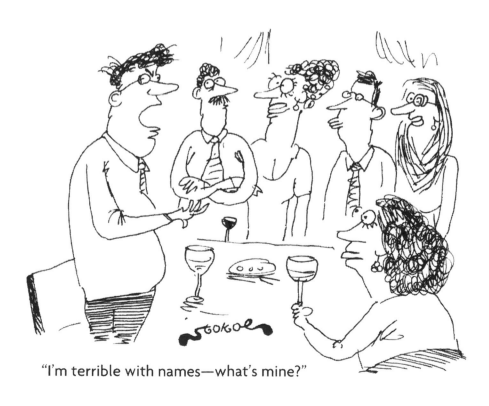

"I'm terrible with names—what's mine?"

215

PEER PRESSURE

What about peer pressure? Sometimes at a party or a gathering well-meaning friends or family members may try to get the individual to eat, which can be uncomfortable. From a psychological perspective, we highly recommend stating that you follow a particular diet and be firm and confident in your resolve. Be aware that anyone who would make fun of you or not encourage you to maintain your diet does not have your best interest in mind.

If the potential embarrassment or peer pressure or desire to eat something is so high that you consume something brain unhealthy, do not freak out! **Even if you completely binge on brain unhealthy foods all night at a particular party, it will not have a large impact as long as you shrug it off and resume your brain-healthy diet the next day.** Remember, part of the challenge to helping one's memory through diet is that the effects will not be immediate. However, the fact that these changes occur over the long-term can also be a benefit. As long as individuals refrain from the dreaded "all-or-nothing-thinking" mentioned earlier, they will succeed in the long run.

SECTION 4

SPECIAL CONSIDERATIONS FOR DIET IN THE TREATMENT OF ALZHEIMER'S DISEASE

CHAPTER 22

How Does Treatment Differ from Prevention?

There have been many studies regarding dietary modification and Alzheimer's disease, and each study has focused on different time points in the course of the disease. For example, some of the studies have asked patients to track the types of foods they eat over long periods of time, and those studies have shown that eating certain foods in moderate to high amounts can have a protective effect on memory loss and dementia. Other studies have specifically focused on dietary changes after a patient has already been diagnosed with AD. For example, some of the highest-quality research in this area was performed by Craft and colleagues, and showed that decreasing carbohydrates and saturated fats can improve memory function in patients with AD. Another excellent study that will be covered later showed that adding a commonly available vitamin can improve effectiveness of some of the medications used for AD.

We now understand that AD "starts" in the brain at least twenty to thirty years before the start of symptoms. This is important because while we do not have clear evidence that many of the dietary interventions that may help to prevent or delay the onset of AD may actually help the symptoms, many physicians still recommend these changes. Even a very slight amount of incremental benefit overtime can possibly help with the course of AD, and as such, the dietary approaches for delaying the onset of AD are essentially quite similar to those used for treatment.

The main difference in nutritional modification for prevention versus treatment lies in the carbohydrate composition of the diet. Individuals already diagnosed with AD may require a more aggressive carbohydrate reducing plan in order to achieve a clinically significant effect. As described earlier in the "Early Bird Special" diet strategy in Chapter 14, the brain may be able to use ketone bodies as an alternative fuel source in the brain (instead of only relying upon glucose, or sugar).

People with AD may also have been diagnosed with other concurrent medical problems, and these need to be taken into consideration. As such, any and all dietary changes need to be made with the approval and supervision of the treating physician. This is important in case the diet strategies being used to promote brain health may not be advisable for certain individuals. For example, certain patients with diabetes (usually type 1 but can also occur with type 2) may be at risk of diabetic ketoacidosis. (See Chapter 18 for symptoms.) These patients would need to avoid dietary changes of very low or no carbohydrates, since this can lead to ketosis and severe health consequences.

CHAPTER 23

Medical Foods in the Treatment of Alzheimer's Disease

A few years ago, the first medical food for Alzheimer's disease was released. This food is supplied as a powder that is mixed with a liquid and consumed after a big meal (breakfast or lunch) once each day.

What is a medical food? This is one of the three categories of pharmacologic agents that physicians may consider for patients with Alzheimer's disease. These three categories include drugs (or medications), supplements (or nutraceuticals), and medical foods.

There are currently four commonly used FDA-approved drugs for the various stages of Alzheimer's disease. While many of us are most familiar with FDA-approved drugs, it is important to review the similarities and differences between each of these therapies.

FDA-APPROVED MEDICATIONS

Prescription drugs are the most well-studied Alzheimer's treatments in terms of effectiveness and safety. The research into these drugs is reviewed by the Food and Drug Administration (FDA), which approves (or denies) the explicit indications for which medications may be used. These Alzheimer's disease–specific claims must be supported by the most comprehensive and well-designed clinical and scientific studies. These studies are pre-approved by the FDA and are designed to highlight potential safety issues. FDA-approved drugs are accompanied by an information sheet called the package insert that contains valuable information. Patients should read and follow the recommendations detailed in the package insert and discuss any questions about drug administration directly with their treating physician.

A prescription drug can make claims of "curing, treating, preventing, or mitigating the effects of symptoms of a specific disease." In order to obtain a drug, patients must get a prescription from their physician and have it filled by a licensed pharmacist.

CURRENTLY USED FDA-APPROVED DRUGS FOR ALZHEIMER'S DISEASE		
BRAND NAME	**SCIENTIFIC NAME**	**RELEASE**
Exelon patch	Rivastigmine	2007
Namenda	Memantine	2003
Razadyne ER	Galantamine	2001
Aricept	Donepezil	1997

SUPPLEMENTS

Dietary supplements, also referred to as nutraceuticals, are products that do not require a prescription from a physician, and are intended to supplement the diet and maintain good health and regular function. Supplements are usually available from a variety of sources, including supermarkets, health food stores, drugstores, and on the Internet. A supplement can contain any one, or a combination of, the following ingredients: vitamins, minerals, herbs or other botanicals, amino acids, dietary substances used to supplement the diet by increasing the total dietary intake (e.g., enzymes from tissues or organs) or a concentrate, metabolite, constituent, or extract.

When looking at the label of any supplement that makes a claim of an effect on structure or function of the body, expect to find the following: "This statement has not been evaluated by the FDA. This product is not intended to diagnose, treat, cure, or prevent any disease."

For additional information, read about the term "dietary supplement" as defined by the Dietary Supplement Health and Education Act (DSHEA) of 1994.

MEDICAL FOOD

As defined by the Orphan Drug Act (1988 Amendment), a medical food is "a food which is formulated to be consumed or administered orally under the supervision of a physician, and which is intended for specific dietary management of a disease or condition for which distinctive nutritional requirements, based on recognized scientific principles, are established by medical evaluation." These therapeutic agents are a heterogeneous group of formulations that comprise a relatively new category of medical protocols defined by Congress and are subject to regulation by the FDA.

Medical foods achieve the "Generally Recognized As

Safe" (GRAS) designation, the highest FDA standard of safety given to foods, which all components of the formulation must satisfy. Additionally, and unlike over-the-counter dietary supplements, they require the supervision and prescription of a physician.

Medical foods and dietary supplements are discrete classifications and are not interchangeable. Medical foods must be shown, by medical evaluation, to meet the distinctive nutritional needs of a specific, diseased patient population being targeted prior to marketing. In contrast, dietary supplements are intended for normal, healthy adults and require no pre-market efficacy tests. In addition, *medical foods require physician supervision and a prescription.*

To summarize, medical foods are medical products for a specific nutritional purpose, as opposed to dietary supplements, which are a consumer product to supplement the diet and maintain good health and regular function.

The name of the medical food product for AD is called Axona, which contains caprylic triglyceride, a medium-chain triglyceride that is broken down by the liver into ketone bodies. It has been known for some time that the brains of patients with AD have a decreased ability to use glucose, and thus ketone bodies may improve cognitive function. Based on the initial study (Henderson, 2009), Axona has been shown to have a positive effect on cognitive function in a specific group of patients (depending on genetic factors). Even more recent evidence shows that roughly 13 percent of APOE4 negative patients may have a dramatic increase in cognitive functioning (also most likely attributable to genetic factors). (See Chapter 15 for information about APOE4.)

Axona is only available with a prescription and must be

used under the supervision of a physician. Since this is a relatively new product, and since medical foods are not commonly used by many physicians, some patients may have difficulty finding a practitioner who is familiar with it. If a patient has difficulty finding a prescriber, there is a list of doctors who have experience with it on the Axona website.

When starting Axona, it is again important to start low and go slow. In Dr. Isaacson's clinical practice, he suggests that his patients start with either a quarter or a half packet per day with food (preferably breakfast or lunch, whichever meal is bigger) for a week and then increase slowly over a week or two to one full packet per day. The powder packet should be mixed with 6–8 ounces of water, meal replacement drink (e.g., Boost), or other liquid (skim milk or juice) to ensure tolerability and must only be taken after a meal.

When the drink is being prepared, it is suggested to first pour 6–8 ounces of liquid into a shaker cup (if a patient gets a sample from their physician, there is usually a shaker cup included), and then the powder added to the liquid. The combination should then be shaken/blended (rather than stirred) to ensure tolerability. It is important to drink the mixture slowly over 20–30 minutes, and the company provides information printed on the sample box that gives helpful hints on how to improve tolerability.

Many patients find it easier to purchase several shaker cups as this will reduce the need to wash them on a daily basis. Some shaker cups come with mixing spheres or "agitators" that help to mix the powder into a more palatable form (purchase these types if possible).

The Axona sample kits that may be available from physicians have miniature packets that contain one-quarter of the full packet amount that is usually dispensed when a patient fills the prescription. The sample kits allow patients to gradually increase the dose of Axona, thus decreasing the likelihood of side effects when first starting the product. If a sample kit is not available and you instead fill a prescription, physicians may suggest starting at a lower dose. Some physicians suggest a quarter of a packet per day for a few days, then a half packet per day for a few days, then three-quarters of a packet per day for a few days, then increasing to the full packet as tolerated. Other physicians may begin at a half a packet per day for a week, then increasing to the full packet. Regardless of how a physician recommends starting Axona, it is imperative to drink the mixture slowly after a big meal (breakfast or lunch) as described above.

Patients who have a history of milk or soy allergies, diabetic ketoacidosis, poorly controlled diabetes, or a variety of other health conditions should not take Axona. This product is generally safe, but as with all therapies, must be used under the close supervision of a physician. As discussed earlier, Axona has been tested in a phase-2 randomized, double-blind, placebo-controlled trial and was shown to be effective for a subset of patients who were negative for the APOE4 gene. While genetic testing is only rarely done by physicians, most prescribers try Axona without ordering genetic testing. If after three months the patient continues to decline, most physicians will stop recommending it. In Dr. Isaacson's clinical practice, he does not yet perform genetic testing for a variety of reasons (which go beyond the scope of this chapter).

The manufacturer has ongoing clinical trials, which are necessary, and more information can also be found online at the FDA clinical trials website (www.clinicaltrials.gov).

Additional information may also be found on the company website. Since Axona is classified as a medical food (and not an FDA-approved drug), some insurance companies may not cover it. In such cases, the manufacture offers a 20 percent discount coupon that may be available on the website (www.about-axona.com) or via the physician's office. The cost (after discount) varies from pharmacy to pharmacy, so it is a good idea to check several. For example, Dr. Isaacson has one patient who pays $72/month, and another who pays $91/month from a different pharmacy in the same city, so it is sensible to check around.

If the future clinical trials are positive, the FDA may review these data and approve Axona as a drug. This would open the door to wider insurance coverage for many individuals.

In clinical practice, physicians tend to suggest that patients engage in a cognitively stimulating activity roughly two hours after drinking Axona. By this time, the ketone bodies have traveled to the brain and may give the brain more "fuel" to participate in activities. For example, one caregiver takes her husband to the movies, and another caregiver listens to the *Therapy for Memory* Music Activity and Educational Program on CD with his wife two hours after administration (see the website resources section at the end of the book, or visit www.therapyformemory.org/music for more information). Social interaction with family or friends is also a great option.

CHAPTER 24

Dietary Modifications for AD Patients with Sleep Difficulties

There are several non-drug dietary options to help manage sleep difficulties. Several of these strategies are easy to implement and may be helpful. The most important is to limit caffeinated beverages and other foods that contain caffeine after lunchtime. It is especially important to avoid caffeine in the afternoon and evening, as this will disrupt sleep 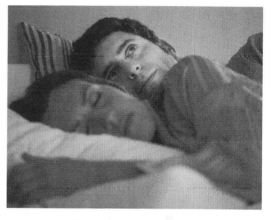 patterns and may make it more difficult for someone to fall asleep.

While coffee is commonly known to contain caffeine, several other foods and beverages may also have significant amounts. For example, most chocolate, coffee-flavored ice creams and candies, teas, sodas, energy-drinks, and certain types of chewing gum may contain caffeine. It is very important to read the nutrition labels on products, and also remember that other additives like ginseng will have a stimulant effect that is similar to that of caffeine.

Also, be careful to monitor over-the-counter medications that may contain stimulants, such as cold and flu products, as these may also affect the sleep-wake cycle. Finally, alcohol intake can have a significant effect on sleep cycles. Having more than a glass of wine before bed to help one sleep may actually be counterproductive over the long haul. Therefore, we recommend avoiding more than one serving of alcohol at night for anyone who has trouble sleeping.

While an in depth discussion on medications for sleep trouble is beyond the scope of this book, there is one specific medication that clinicians may tend to use more than others for patients with AD. This medication is called trazodone (Desyrel), which can be given in low doses before bedtime. This medication needs to be prescribed by and used under the supervision of a qualified medical professional. One of the strategies that physicians also use is to avoid is the use of sedative medications in AD patients. These medications, which are in the category called benzodiazepines, are commonly known as diazepam (Valium), lorazepam (Ativan), and clonazepam (Klonopin), as well as similar medications such as zolpidem (Ambien).

Using the strategy of "start low, go slow" is helpful with these medications. For trazodone, some will most commonly start with 25 mg about 30 minutes before bedtime (sometimes starting lower at 12.5 mg, particularly in older patients), and use this dose for at least a few days or up to a week before making an increase. If the medication is not helpful after a week or so, it can be increased to 50 mg before bedtime, as tolerated. Continued reassessment is important, and the maximum dose is quite variable depending upon the patient and severity of disease. Other agents that may be considered include eszopiclone (Lunesta) and ramelton (Rozerem). Some clinicians use Lunesta with caution as it is also a benzodiazepine receptor agonist and has a longer half-life, possibly worsening the "hangover effect" on cognition in the morning. Others have used mirtazapine (Remeron) instead, which can help sleep at low doses of 7.5 mg each evening. At low doses, Remeron is generally well tolerated but at higher doses, adverse effects may occur (e.g., weight gain).

Daytime bright-light exposure is postulated to strengthen (increase the amplitude) of the circadian (biological-clock driven) sleep-wake rhythm. This is also a helpful recommendation that may be considered, and in addition to sunlight, portable and at-home light boxes are now available for purchase. A new study by Figuiero and colleagues published in the *Journal of Alzheimer's Disease* showed that tailored light exposure is a viable therapeutic option for reducing sleep disturbances in patients with AD. This was the first study to demonstrate that those who experienced lower levels of light exposure during the day also had lower activity levels, and had greater disruption of the natural sleep or "circadian" rhythms. This was greatest in the winter months. While we do not yet know the best amount of light exposure to help, therapy could range from going outdoors for 10–15 each day to sitting in front of a light box (fitted with blue LEDs) for a prescribed amount of time during the day. Visit www.TheADplan.com/blog/worpress to learn more.

CHAPTER 25

Increasing the Effectiveness of AD Medications with Dietary Modification and Vitamins

In Dr. Isaacson's clinical practice, he almost always starts the vitamin folic acid 1 mg with a cholinesterase inhibitor (Aricept [donepezil], Exelon patch [rivastigmine] and Razadyne [galantamine]) in his patients. A small research study showed increased clinical benefit of the cholinesterase medications when folic acid was used in combination (*International Journal of Geriatric Psychiatry*, 2008). While this study needs to be repeated, we do tend to recommend the addition of folic acid because it is relatively safe. Foods high in folic acid, including dark leafy greens, citrus fruits, and broccoli, should also be considered as part of a brain-healthy diet. Like all interventions, adding this vitamin or increasing intake of these foods should be discussed with and approved by the treating physician.

Another way to ensure optimal effectiveness of drugs is to take them as directed (e.g., with or after a meal, as directed by the physician) and try not to miss any doses. Missing doses for several days or several weeks can have a significant negative effect. In fact, in several of Dr. Isaacson's patients, re-starting the medications after not taking them for many weeks did not bring the patient back to the same level as before he or she stopped taking them. We thus advocate for the caregiver and patient to work together to ensure that doses are not missed. When necessary, a home healthcare nurse may be suggested by the treating physician. The nurse will make periodic home visits to help with medication administration and record keeping.

In the future, the area of personalized nutrition and nutrigenomics (see Chapter 15 for more details) should expand, and researchers should learn additional strategies to improve medication effectiveness. Until that time, it is important to combine several dietary strategies along with medications, physical exercise, mental stimulation (like music activity and educational programs) and social stimulation, since these may all synergize together to provide additional benefits.

CHAPTER 26

Decreasing Side Effects of AD Medications with Dietary Modification

Several medications indicated for AD may cause side effects if not taken appropriately. For each of the cholinesterase inhibitor medications (Aricept [donepezil], Exelon patch [rivastigmine] and Razadyne [galantamine]), if side effects occur when the dose has been first started or has been increased, the treating physician may suggest decreasing the dose. Medications like Aricept and Razadyne are usually tolerated better when given with a big meal (breakfast or lunch, whichever meal is bigger). Since the Exelon patch is absorbed by the body through the skin over a 24-hour period, it is less important to eat a full meal when the patch is placed; however, eating regular healthy meals throughout the day is advised to ensure tolerability.

There are currently three dosages available for the Exelon patch, with the most recent dose of 13.3 mg released in October 2012. It is important to use this medication as directed and patients should always be started first on 4.6 mg each day for four weeks, and then increasing it to the 9.5 mg dose if tolerated. While the 4.6 mg dose of the Exelon patch may be sufficient for patients who weigh less than 110 pounds and those with other medical conditions (this decision should be discussed with the treating physician), Dr. Isaacson increases to the 9.5 mg dose in most of his patients. Occasionally, if a patient is unable to tolerate the 9.5 mg patch, based on the clinical trial data, the lower 4.6 mg dose of the Exelon patch may not be sufficient to provide a therapeutic benefit. In this case, the treating physician may switch to an alternative medication. If the 9.5 mg patch is tolerated, the treating physician may decide to increase to the 13.3 mg patch as tolerated.

With Aricept, if side effects are experienced when either starting the medication or increasing the dose, it is important to ensure that the dose was taken correctly (with a big meal, either breakfast or lunch). It is preferable to have some healthy fat in the meal as this may increase tolerability. If side effects occur after starting the 5 mg dose, a re-trial at 2.5 mg with food may be suggested by the physician. If side effects occur after increasing to the 10 mg dose, reducing the dose back down to 5 mg may be suggested for a few days, and a re-trial of 7.5 mg (one and a half tablets of 5 mg) may be considered in the future instead of increasing to 10 mg. If the treating physician suggests a subsequent increase to 23 mg, it may be best tolerated after at least three months on the 10 mg dose, and after a big meal. There have been several reports of increased side effects on the 23 mg dose, so patients should discuss this with the treating physician and again, take with a big meal earlier in the day.

With Razadyne ER, if a side effect is experienced with the 16 mg or 24 mg per day dose, it is again important to ensure that the dose was taken correctly (with a big meal, either breakfast or lunch). The minimum therapeutic dose is 16 mg per day and as such, if a patient can only tolerate the 8 mg per day dose, the treating physician may decide to switch to different medication in this category.

In general, if a side effect occurs with any of these treatments, doses may be skipped or drug dosage reduced until the negative effects disappear, and a higher dosage may be tried again at a later date. Positive effects on memory, thinking skills, functioning of everyday activities, and behavior may be countered by adverse side effects such as nausea, vomiting, and diarrhea, which also become more likely with dosage increases. It is important to find a favorable balance between side effects and the overall effectiveness of the medication. Other side effects like a slow heart rate and weight loss can also occur, so these need to be reported to and reviewed by the treating physician.

If patients do not tolerate one cholinesterase inhibitor, they may tolerate another, so the treating physician may consider a switch. Also, if one cholinesterase inhibitor is not effective or the patient continues to decline, the physician may consider switching to an alternative medication.

Conclusion

The overall goal of *The Alzheimer's Diet* is to provide the tools and resources necessary for anyone to make adjustments to their diet to help protect and support their memory for the rest of their life. Central to this is a focus on adjusting dietary habits over time and looking at this plan as making slow but steady life-long changes rather than as "going on a diet."

The more brain-healthy foods (and the fewer brain-*un*healthy foods) eaten, the better. But always remember, this is not an all-or-nothing plan. Everyone has days where they eat more or fewer healthy foods and that is okay, as long as a continual effort is made to make better choices.

Although we provide very detailed descriptions and instructions in *The Alzheimer's Diet*, the essential element of this program is for people to try different strategies to discover what works for them. With education about what foods can help versus harm the brain, and making smart choices, everyone can improve their overall brain health!

Both this book and the AD-NTS were developed to provide the tools to make this possible. While we hope we have accomplished our goals to educate and inform you about why and how to use diet and nutrition to fight AD and memory loss, please let us know how we did! Visit the website below to rate your experience with this book and provide feedback, as well as offer suggestions for future editions. Your time and input are greatly appreciated!

READER SURVEY

To complete a reader survey about this book, and earn a chance at a $100 Amazon.com gift certificate, please visit www.AlzheimersDiet.com/Survey.

Helpful Websites
for Patients and Caregivers

www.TheADplan.com
New book by Dr. Isaacson on the latest advances in the
treatment and prevention of AD, including medications,
vitamins, lifestyle changes, and diet.

Also available in Spanish
(www.TheADplan.com/Espanol)

www.TherapyForMemory.org
Current Information on How to Fight Memory Loss,
Ask the Experts Section, and Doctor-Recommended
Brain Stimulating Activities (like the new Music Activity
and Educational Program on CD and Tranquil
Sounds for Relaxation and Sleep CD)

www.alz.org
Caregiver Resources, Support Groups and Information
and Educational Opportunities about AD

www.alzfdn.org
Information and Resources about AD for
Patients/Families

www.health.gov
Helpful Educational Information about Health
and Nutrition

www.nia.nih.gov/alzheimers
Excellent Overview of AD by National Institutes
of Health

www.lumosity.com
Brain Activity Program to Use Weekly and
Track Progress

www.AlzRisk.org
Provides a comprehensive, unbiased, centralized,
publicly available and regularly updated collection
of epidemiologic reports that evaluate environmental
(i.e., non-genetic) risk factors for AD in well-defined
study populations. Database can be searched by a variety
of dropdown menus or by specific keywords. For each
risk factor, tables of all research studies are provided.

Food Terminology

Artificial Sweeteners: Do not affect blood sugar levels but are made of synthetic compounds. While there is ongoing controversy over whether artificial sweeteners pose health risks, the FDA has not been presented with sufficient scientific evidence to deem them unsafe. There is, however, some evidence to suggest that beverages with artificial sweeteners may become hazardous if kept at elevated temperatures (above 80°F) for several days. Further study is indeed warranted.

Bran: The covering or outer part of the grain, which contains the highest concentration of fiber, B vitamins, and antioxidants.

"Cage-free" Eggs: The U.S. Department of Agriculture requires only that hens spend part of their time outside in order for producers to label them as "cage-free" or "free-range" eggs. It is important to note that "cage-free" does not necessarily imply "organic." Organic eggs are from hens fed organic feed and not given antibiotics. Organic eggs are frequently higher in omega-3 fatty acids, making them a healthier option relative to regular (and most cage-free) eggs.

Egg Substitutes: Made with egg whites, which usually have 0 mg of cholesterol ($^1/_4$ cup) versus over 200 mg in one equivalently sized large egg. Some brands contain up to 99 percent of egg whites, along with a mixture of dairy products, vegetable gums, vitamins, and other nutrients. The refrigerated Egg Beaters Original is one example to be considered.

Enriched vs. Fortified: *Enriched* refers to replacement of lost nutrients after processing. This includes the vitamins folic acid, iron, niacin, riboflavin, and thiamine, often necessary to meet FDA standards. When making food choices, enriched foods indicate that the food has been processed, thereby losing nutrients. Avoid this type of processed food when possible, and preferentially choose fresh (or raw) food, either with or without fortified nutrients. *Fortified* refers to nutrients that are added to the food, in addition to the nutrients that were in the food originally. However, this does not necessarily make them a healthier option relative to fresh foods.

Extra-Virgin Olive Oil: Produced from pressing the olives without the addition of solvents. Must have low free-acidity (less than 0.8 percent), which indicates higher quality. Still high in total fat and calories (so use small amounts) but shown to raise HDL ("good") cholesterol.

"Excellent Source of," "High," "Rich in": Contains at least 20 percent of the Daily Value of a specific nutrient *or* type of dietary fiber.

Fresh Food: No processing, preservation, or freezing. Also referred to as raw food.

Glycemic Index: Classification system to indicate the relative blood glucose response to carbohydrate-containing foods. It is a ranking on a scale from 0 to 100 of carbohydrates according to the extent to which they raise blood glucose levels (and subsequently, how much insulin is released by the body as a response). Low-glycemic index foods produce less of a pronounced increase in blood glucose and insulin levels, likely due to their slow metabolism, digestion, and/or absorption. High-glycemic index foods require more insulin to metabolize and cause a more pronounced increase in blood glucose.

High-Fructose Corn Syrup (HFCS): While having the same relative sweetness as fructose, it is highly processed and, most important, has a high-glycemic index. Despite associated health concerns (e.g., obesity, metabolic syndrome), corn syrup has become widespread due to the lower cost relative refined sugar, prolongation of shelf life, and ease of mixing in beverages.

Minimally Processed Natural Sweeteners: A variety of sweeteners derived from plants. Some of the more recent and popular choices include agave nectar, stevia, and raw (unfiltered) honey. Others include unsulfured blackstrap molasses, raw dried dates/date sugar, and 100 percent pure dark maple syrup. These types of sweeteners have somewhat of a "stronger" taste, so the same desired sweetness can be achieved by using less of it, thereby reducing caloric intake, blood glucose, and insulin release.

Monounsaturated Fat: Sometimes called the "heart-healthy fat," which can actually reduce the "bad" cholesterol (LDL).

"Omega-3" Eggs: Hens are fed diet rich in omega-3 fatty acids (e.g., flaxseeds, alpha-linolenic acid). Look for brands with at least 200 mg per egg.

Organic: Certified to be produced by certain standards (e.g., handling, storage, production) and ingredients are free from prohibited substances (e.g., synthetic pesticides, chemical fertilizers) and are not genetically modified. In the United States production is managed via the Organic Foods Production Act (OFPA), which integrates cultural, biological, and mechanical methods that foster "cycling of resources, promote ecological balance, and conserve biodiversity."

Polyunsaturated Fat: Contains a balance of omega-3 and omega-6 fatty acids.

Processed: Any food that has been altered or changed from its natural state. This may occur due to convenience (e.g., storage or packaging) or for safety reasons (e.g., pasteurization of milk and orange juice, which is a process to kill bacteria). Not all processed foods are "bad" per se, but often when foods are canned, frozen, or dehydrated, some of the "good" nutrients are lost, and some "bad" ingredients are added.

Refined Sugar: Sugar that has gone through the process of extracting the sugar (sucrose) from the plant materials and then removing other unwanted materials from the extracted raw sugar (e.g., stalk fibers from the sugar cane or sugar beets). Completely refined white sugar is nearly 100 percent sucrose and essentially contains no nutritional elements (e.g., vitamins, minerals, proteins), accounting for expressions like "empty calories" or "junk food." In the last few years, a new refined sugar with a lower glycemic index was released in Australia. Per the company website, LoGiCane is less refined than white, raw, and brown sugar and retains many of the nutrients usually washed out in processing (e.g., polyphenols, antioxidants, organic minerals, and calcium).

Saturated Fat: High intake is linked to heart disease, obesity, and some cancers. Can raise LDL cholesterol (the "bad" cholesterol). There are a number of saturated fats; some are safer than others. In general, however, it is a good idea to limit saturated fats.

Sugar Alcohols: Also known as polyols, these are less sweet than sugar, have fewer calories, and have a lower glycemic index.

Sugar Substitutes: Simulate the taste of sugar, have fewer calories (energy), and can be made out of natural or synthetic components. Six are currently approved for use in the U.S. (five synthetic: aspartame, sucralose, neotame, acesulfame potassium, saccharin; one natural: stevia).

Trans Fat: Linked to obesity, heart disease, accelerated aging, and cancer. Difficult for the body to break down. Be aware that foods that advertise having "no trans fat" may still be high in saturated (and/ or unsaturated) fat and calories. In addition, FDA regulations allow food processors to claim "zero trans fats" on the label even if the food actually contains 0.49 grams (per serving). If the ingredients are examined, individuals may notice partially hydrogenated oil, which is the primary source of trans fat.

Whole Grain: Contains all of the naturally occurring elements, such as the bran, endosperm (e.g., starchy carbohydrates, protein), and germ. Whole wheat is a form of whole grain. Wheat is just one (healthy) form of grain. The important thing is to look for "whole" on the packaging (or first ingredient), and avoid "multi-grain" or "seven-grain," as these may still not contain the most healthy parts of the grains.

Brain-Healthy
Food Substitution Guide

Do you usually start the day with cereal, instant oatmeal, or white toast? Try non-fat plain yogurt (no sugar added), berries/nuts, steal-cut oats, or egg-white omelet with broccoli, spinach, and non-fat shredded cheese.

Two packets of sugar in your coffee? Try decreasing to one and a half, and then again to one packet (or less!), slowly over time so that your taste buds can accommodate. Or try minimally processed natural sweeteners, like agave nectar, a touch of honey (raw, unfiltered), or stevia (natural sugar substitute) instead.

Only have cranberry, orange, or apple juice in the refrigerator? Fill half the cup with water, add ice, and then fill the rest up with juice. Better yet, drink a full glass of water first at the start of the meal.

In the cereal aisle at the supermarket? Choose cereals high in fiber (greater than 6 gm/serving), which helps to slow digestion and reduce sugar/insulin level fluctuations in the blood. All-Bran (Extra Fiber) and Kashi (Go Lean) are two to consider.

Used to having a sandwich for lunch? Try a salad instead, adding lean turkey or grilled chicken breast, with berries, avocado, chickpeas, beans, berries, flaxseeds, and a drizzle of extra virgin olive oil, fat-free balsamic, or raspberry vinaigrette.

Can't say no to bread? Say yes to 100 percent whole grain, containing at least a few grams of fiber per serving.

Craving French fries? Replace with oven-baked sweet potato fries.

Cheese, please? Try fat-free cheddar, Swiss, cream, or cottage cheese.

Soups on? Gazpacho, miso broth, or vegetable with cubes of turkey, chicken, or tofu.

Prefer sweetened iced tea? Start by adding half as much sweetener as usual, then reduce the amount added gradually over several weeks until your taste buds accommodate. Or try minimally processed natural sweeteners, like agave nectar or a small amount of honey (raw, unfiltered) instead.

Eating a heavy dinner? Add some vinegar to your salad before the meal, which may help to delay digestion, thereby reducing glycemic index.

Dining out? Look for the health-conscious menu—most restaurants (even fast food) have several options on the menu.

Pasta night? Try spaghetti squash, or a small serving of 100 percent whole grain (e.g., whole wheat) pasta, cooked firm, which lowers glycemic index.

Think white rice is nice? How about brown rice (e.g., brown Basmati), quinoa, couscous, or barley instead.

In the mood for mashed potatoes? Try mashed cauliflower instead. Other root vegetables like celery root or turnips work too.

An alcoholic drink with dinner? A daily glass of red (or white) wine may be good for the heart and brain.

Need a snack between meals, can't say no to dessert, or no time for a full meal since you are on the go? Try a small handful of nuts (due to fat content, should be consumed in moderation), or fruit instead, like berries, or better yet a smoothie (with fresh fruits and vegetables, no added sugar and non-fat milk or yogurt).

Chocoholic? Small amounts of dark chocolate, low-carb, sugar-free, or sweetened with sugar alcohols may be best (e.g., mannitol, sorbitol).

Brain-Healthy Menu Options

EXAMPLE DAILY MENUS FOR BRAIN-HEALTHY EATING

MONDAY	
Breakfast	Scrambled eggs. 3 egg whites or egg substitute, scrambled in a little skim milk, with chopped fresh tomato, onion, and spinach. Serve with 1 slice rye toast. Black or green tea or coffee.
Lunch	Tuna or chicken lettuce wrap. Mix tuna or chunked chicken with fat-free mayonnaise and raisins. Wrap in full piece lettuce.
Snack	Chips and salsa dip. Flaxseed tortilla chips. Mix $1/2$ cup salsa with fresh avocado and 1 tbsp fat-free sour cream.
Dinner	Flatbread pepperoni pizza (see Chapter 9 for recipe). 1 glass concord grape juice.
Dessert	Cinnamon baked apples. Sliced apples baked with cinnamon, small amount raw honey, topped with Kashi GoLean Crunch.

TUESDAY	
Breakfast	Pancakes. Whole-wheat or flaxseed pancakes sweetened with sucralose and/or applesauce (no sugar added). Add blueberries, raspberries, and strawberries. Use cooking spray on the pan. Up to 2 tbsp maple syrup if desired. Black or green tea or coffee.
Lunch	Boca burger (see Chapter 9 for recipe).
Snack	Trail mix with peanuts, almonds, raisins, and dried apricots.

| Dinner | Chicken with balsamic fig sauce (see Appendix E for recipe). 1 glass concord grape juice. |
| Dessert | Cupcakes. Make with steel-cut oats, peanut butter, blueberries, protein or cocoa powder, and sugar-free sweetener. |

WEDNESDAY	
Breakfast	Egg-white western omelet. 3 egg whites or egg substitute with fat free cheese and spinach, topped with salsa, and made with cooking spray. One-third cup black or baked beans. Black or green tea or coffee.
Lunch	Tuna and soup. Half tuna-salad sandwich made with fat-free mayonnaise on 1 slice rye toast. Bowl of low sodium chicken, vegetable, lentil or split-pea soup.
Snack	Hummus with raw vegetables, such as carrots, broccoli, and cauliflower.
Dinner	Herbed steak (see Appendix E for recipe). 1 glass red wine.
Dessert	Hot fudge sundae (see Chapter 9 for recipe).

THURSDAY	
Breakfast	Fruit smoothie. Blend $1/2$ cup strawberries and blueberries with $1/2$ cup Greek yogurt and $1/3$ cup ice. Add 2 tsp nonnutritive sweetener. Black or green tea or coffee.
Lunch	Spinach salad. Fresh spinach with chunks of chicken, walnuts, and pomegranate seeds. Fat-free balsamic vinaigrette dressing.
Snack	Protein bar (see Chapter 6 for optimum brain-healthy criteria).
Dinner	Grilled rosemary salmon skewers (see Appendix E for recipe). 1 glass concord grape juice.
Dessert	Strawberries 'n cream. Chopped strawberries with $1/2$ cup fat-free half and half. Add small amount sucralose to desired sweetness.

FRIDAY	
Breakfast	Poached egg with barley and spinach (see Appendix E for recipe). Black or green tea or coffee.
Lunch	Moo shu chicken (see Appendix E for recipe).
Snack	Large apple and $1/2$ cup pumpkin seeds.
Dinner	Antipasto. Whole-wheat pasta with chopped broccoli, carrots, zucchini, and arugula. Add 2 tbsp extra virgin olive oil, 2 tbsp balsamic vinegar, 2 tbsp cooking wine, and $1/4$ cup grated parmesan cheese. 1 glass red wine.
Dessert	Fruit, nut, and chocolate cup. Top 1 cup blueberries, raspberries, and strawberries with 1 tablespoon dark-chocolate chips and 1 tablespoon chopped nuts.

SATURDAY	
Breakfast	Oatmeal. Rolled oat oatmeal with blueberries, nonnutritive sweetener. Black or green tea or coffee.
Lunch	Citrus-chili shrimp (see Appendix E for recipe).
Snack	Fruit salad and nuts. 1 cup fruit salad. $1/3$ cup of dry roasted almonds, hazelnuts, walnuts, pecans, pistachios, cashews, or macadamia nuts.
Dinner	Grilled salmon. Large grilled salmon steak topped with 2 tbsp mango salsa, served with asparagus and $1/3$ cup whole grain brown rice. 1 glass red wine.
Dessert	Chocolate indulgence. 2 oz 90-percent cocoa dark chocolate (approximately $1/2$ bar). 1 cup skim milk with cocoa powder.

SUNDAY	
Breakfast	Berry and flaxseed breakfast smoothie (see Appendix E for recipe). Black or green tea or coffee.
Lunch	Lentil soup. Low-sodium lentil soup with $1/2$ cup chunks of chicken or ham added. 1 slice rye toast.
Snack	Peanut butter muffin. Spread 1 tbsp natural no-sugar-added peanut butter on whole-grain toast or English muffin.
Dinner	Curry chicken. Prepare with extra virgin olive oil. Serve with whole-grain brown rice. 1 glass concord grape juice.
Dessert	Sundae Top. 3 tbsp fat-free whip cream with $1/2$ cup raspberries and blackberries on top. Add $1/4$ cup nuts if desired.

GENERAL GUIDELINES FOR BRAIN-HEALTHY DIET (PERCENT DAILY INTAKE):

Include the following suggested breakdown of macronutrients (modified from Craft study):

- Fat: 25 percent (less than 7 percent of which saturated)

- Carbohydrates: 30–45 percent (low-glycemic index)

- Protein: 25–35 percent

Sample Recipes

BREAKFAST

Berries and Flaxseed Smoothie

Servings:
1 smoothie

Prep Time:
5 minutes

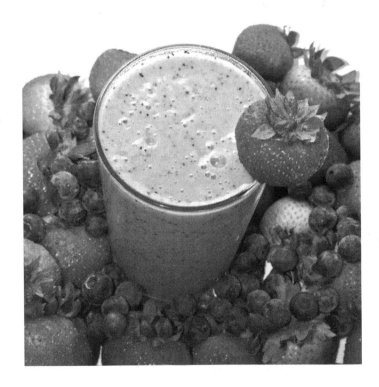

1 cup frozen berries (blueberries, blackberries, raspberries, and/or strawberries)

1 scoop whey protein powder

1 tablespoon ground flaxseed

2 teaspoons lemon juice

1 teaspoon unsweetened cranberry juice

1 Stevia packet

8 ice cubes

$1/2$ cup nonfat Greek yogurt (vanilla)

$1/2$ cup water

Directions:

In a blender, blend all ingredients until smooth. Adjust amount of water for desired thickness.

NUTRITION FACTS

Serving Size 515 g	
Amount Per Serving	
Calories 200	Calories from Fat 38
	% Daily Value
Total Fat 5g	**8%**
Saturated Fat 0.0g	
Trans Fat 0.0g	
Cholesterol 2mg	
Sodium 125mg	**5%**
Total Carbohydrates 23g	**8%**
Dietary Fiber 7.0g	**28%**
Sugars 13g	
Protein 26g	

Poached Egg with Barley and Spinach

Servings: 1

Prep time:
5 minutes
(not counting
barley prep
time)

Cook time:
16–18 minutes

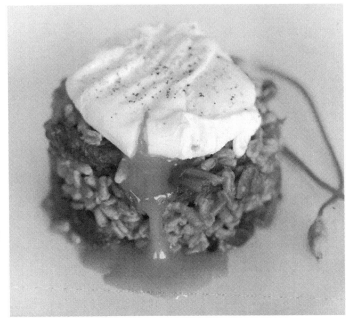

95 g chopped frozen spinach,
thawed and drained

1 g cooking spray (= 1-second spray)

1 large egg

$1/_4$ cup cooked barley

1 teaspoon fat free heavy cream or half & half

$1/_8$ teaspoon garlic powder

Dash sea salt

Dash freshly ground black pepper

Directions:

1. Preheat oven to 400° F.

2. Grease a small cup with 1 squirt cooking spray. Put spinach in a small bowl and blend with garlic powder, salt, and pepper. Lightly pack the spinach and barley in the cup and make an indentation in the center with a tablespoon.

3. Crack the egg into another cup, keeping the yolk whole. Gently pour on top of spinach and cover evenly with fat-free heavy cream.

4. Bake for 16–18 minutes, depending upon desired doneness.

NUTRITION FACTS

Serving Size 158 g	
Amount Per Serving	
Calories 135	Calories from Fat 45
	% Daily Value
Total Fat 5g	**8%**
Saturated Fat 1.5g	**8%**
Trans Fat 0.0g	
Cholesterol 145mg	**57%**
Sodium 135mg	**6%**
Total Carbohydrates 14g	**5%**
Dietary Fiber 6.0g	**24%**
Sugars 6g	
Protein 17g	

LUNCH

Moo Shu Chicken

Servings: 4

Prep time:
5 minutes

Cook time:
8–15 minutes

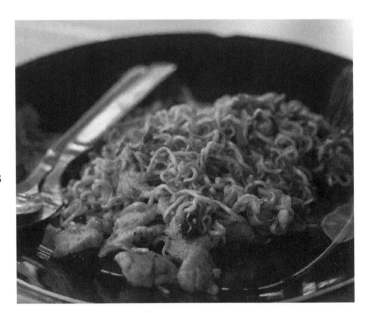

MARINADE:

1 tablespoon low-sodium soy sauce

1 tablespoon sesame oil

1 clove garlic, crushed

1 teaspoon grated fresh ginger

$1/_2$ teaspoon Chinese Five Spice powder

Stir-Fry:

1 pound boneless chicken, cut into $1/2$-inch strips

2 medium stalks celery, thinly sliced

3 cloves crushed garlic

1 tablespoon grated fresh ginger

6 ounces fresh shitake mushrooms,
sliced into $1/2$-inch strips

1 cup sliced green onion (scallions) (about 6 onions)

4 cups sliced cabbage ($1/2$-inch strips)

8 ounces bean sprouts (mung beans are good,
or any type intended for stir-frying)

1 tablespoon low-sodium soy sauce

1 teaspoon extra-virgin olive oil

1 g cooking spray

Directions:

1. Mix together marinade ingredients, add chicken, and mix to coat.

2. Prepare vegetables, and grate ginger and garlic. Heat large skillet on medium-high heat with oil and cooking spray.

3. Add the chicken, and stir-fry until just cooked through (3–4 minutes). Then remove chicken from pan.

4. Add the sesame oil, celery, ginger, and garlic, and sauté for 1 minute.

5. Add mushrooms, onions, cabbage, and bean sprouts in that order, and stir-fry for 1–2 minutes after each.

6. Add the soy sauce and the chicken, and toss to combine.

NUTRITION FACTS

Serving Size 347 g

Amount Per Serving

Calories 300   Calories from Fat 67

                                                              % Daily Value

Total Fat 8g	**12%**
Saturated Fat 1.5g	**8%**
Trans Fat 0.0g	
Cholesterol 57mg	**19%**
Sodium 435mg	**22%**
Total Carbohydrates 17g	**6%**
Dietary Fiber 5g	**20%**
Sugars 5.4g	
Protein 38g	

Citrus-Chili Shrimp

Servings: 4

Prep time:
15 minutes

Cook time:
15 minutes

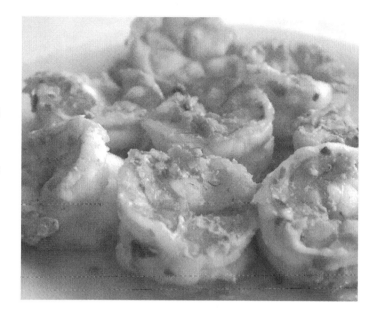

$^1/_8$ cup plus 1 teaspoon extra-virgin olive oil, divided

$^1/_3$ cup fresh orange juice, divided

2 tablespoons grated orange rind

1 tablespoon fresh lime juice

$^1/_2$ teaspoon salt

$^1/_4$ teaspoon red pepper flakes

$^1/_4$ teaspoon chili powder

$^1/_4$ teaspoon ground cumin

1 pound jumbo shrimp, peeled and deveined

1 teaspoon butter substitute
(e.g., I can't believe it's not butter)

Directions:

1. In a bowl, mix $^1/_8$ cup olive oil, 3 tablespoons orange juice, orange rind, lime juice, salt, red pepper, chili powder, and cumin.

2. Add shrimp and marinate 10 minutes.

3. In a large skillet over high heat, melt butter substitute with remaining teaspoon of olive oil.

4. Remove shrimp from marinade; reserve marinade.

5. Add shrimp to skillet and cook for approximately 4 minutes until no longer pink and just cooked through.

6. Transfer shrimp to a serving plate.

7. Add reserved marinade and remaining orange juice to skillet, and boil for 1 minute. Then drizzle over shrimp.

NUTRITION FACTS

Serving Size 155 g	
Amount Per Serving	
Calories 160	Calories from Fat 55
	% Daily Value
Total Fat 7g	**10%**
Saturated Fat 1.3g	**6%**
Trans Fat 0.0g	
Cholesterol 48mg	**17%**
Sodium 470mg	**24%**
Total Carbohydrates 3.4g	**1%**
Dietary Fiber 1g	**4%**
Sugars 2g	
Protein 18.5g	

Chicken with Balsamic Fig Sauce

Servings: 4

Prep time:
5 minutes

Cook time:
18 minutes

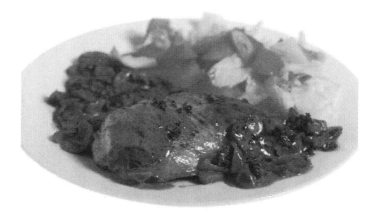

4 (6-ounce) skinless, boneless chicken breast halves

1 1/2 tablespoons fresh thyme leaves, divided

1/2 teaspoon salt, divided

1/4 teaspoon freshly ground black pepper

1 teaspoon olive oil

I teaspoon butter substitute

3/4 cup chopped onion

1/2 cup fat-free, low-sodium chicken broth

1/4 cup balsamic vinegar

2 teaspoon low-sodium soy sauce

1/2 cup finely chopped dried figs (such as Mission)

Directions:

1. Sprinkle both sides of chicken evenly with $1^1/_2$ teaspoons thyme, $^1/_4$ teaspoon salt, and pepper. Heat oil in a large nonstick skillet over medium-high heat. Add chicken; cook 6 minutes on each side or until done. Remove from pan; keep warm.

2. Reduce heat to medium; add butter substitute to pan. Add onion; sauté 3 minutes.

3. Add broth, vinegar, soy sauce, and figs. Simmer until sauce is reduced to 1 cup (about 3 minutes).

4. Add 1 tablespoon thyme and $^1/_4$ teaspoon salt. Cut chicken breast halves lengthwise on the diagonal into slices. Serve sauce over chicken.

NUTRITION FACTS

Serving Size 268 g	
Amount Per Serving	
Calories 282	Calories from Fat 39
	% Daily Value
Total Fat 5g	**8%**
Saturated Fat 1g	**5%**
Trans Fat 0.0g	
Cholesterol 76mg	**24%**
Sodium 452mg	**23%**
Total Carbohydrates 18g	**6%**
Dietary Fiber 3.2g	**14%**
Sugars 13g	
Protein 36.4g	

DINNER

Grilled Rosemary Salmon Skewers

Servings: 4

Prep time:
20 minutes

Cook time:
10 minutes

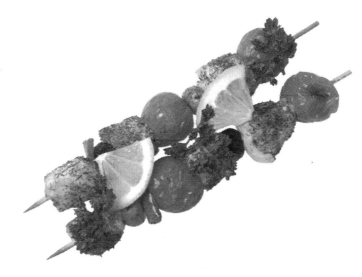

2 teaspoon minced fresh rosemary

1 teaspoon extra-virgin olive oil

2 cloves garlic, minced

1 teaspoon freshly grated lemon zest

1 teaspoon lemon juice

$1/2$ teaspoon kosher salt

$1/4$ teaspoon freshly ground pepper

1 pound center-cut salmon fillet,
skinned and cut into 1-inch cubes

1 pint cherry tomatoes

Directions:

1. Preheat grill to medium-high.

2. Combine rosemary, oil, garlic, lemon zest, lemon juice, salt, and pepper in a medium bowl. Add salmon; toss to coat. Alternating the salmon and tomatoes, divide among eight 12-inch skewers.

3. Oil the grill rack. Grill the kebab, carefully turning once, until the salmon is cooked through, 4 to 6 minutes total. Serve immediately.

NUTRITION FACTS

Serving Size 194 g	
Amount Per Serving	
Calories 190	Calories from Fat 45
	% Daily Value
Total Fat 5.2g	8%
Saturated Fat 1g	5%
Trans Fat 0.0g	
Cholesterol 56mg	20%
Sodium 235mg	12%
Total Carbohydrates 4g	1%
Dietary Fiber 1.2g	5%
Sugars 2g	
Protein 30g	

Herbed Steak

Servings: 4

Prep time:
5 minutes

Cook time:
15–20 minutes

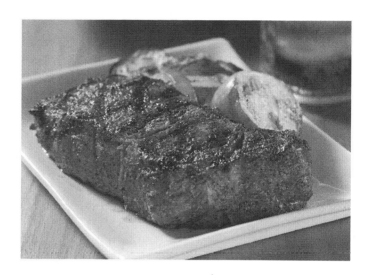

1 teaspoon cracked black pepper

2 teaspoon dried Italian seasoning, crushed

1 teaspoon garlic powder

$^1/_4$ teaspoon salt

2 boneless beef top loin steaks, cut $^3/_4$-inch thick

1 tablespoon extra-virgin olive oil

$^1/_2$ cup reduced-sodium beef broth

1 tablespoon balsamic vinegar

1 tablespoon butter substitute

2 tablespoon snipped fresh flat-leaf parsley

Directions:

1. Combine cracked pepper, Italian seasoning, garlic powder, and salt in a small bowl. Sprinkle evenly over both sides of each steak; rub in with your fingers.

2. Squirt a small amount of cooking spray into a heavy large skillet over medium fire. Add steaks; cook until desired doneness, turning once halfway through cooking time. Allow 10 to 13 minutes for medium-rare doneness (145°F) to medium doneness (160°F). Remove steaks from skillet, reserving drippings in the skillet. Keep steaks warm.

3. For sauce, carefully add beef broth and balsamic vinegar to the skillet; stir to scrape up any crusty brown bits from bottom of skillet. Bring to boiling. Boil gently, uncovered, about 4 minutes or until sauce is reduced by half. Remove from heat; stir in butter substitute.

4. Divide sauce among 4 dinner plates. Cut each steak in half. Place a piece of meat on top of sauce on each plate; sprinkle with parsley.

NUTRITION FACTS

Serving Size 90 g	
Amount Per Serving	
Calories 171	Calories from Fat 50
	% Daily Value
Total Fat 5.9g	9%
Saturated Fat 1.8g	7%
Trans Fat 0.0g	
Cholesterol 47mg	17%
Sodium 335mg	14%
Total Carbohydrates 1.4g	0%
Dietary Fiber 1.0g	4%
Sugars 0.6g	
Protein 21.7g	

9-Week Diet Plan Nutrition Tracking Log Sheets

All information can be entered online using the AD-NTS

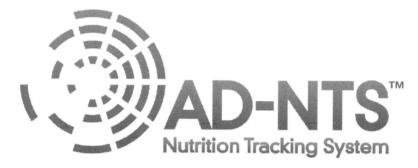

www.AlzheimersDiet.com

WEEK 1	
TOTAL GRAMS OF CARBOHYDRATES	
Sun:	Thurs:
Mon:	Fri:
Tue:	Sat:
Wed:	

3 FAVORITE BRAIN-UNHEALTHY SNACKS AND
3 FAVORITE BRAIN UNHEALTHY MEALS:

Brain-*unhealthy* Snacks

1.

2.

3.

Brain-*unhealthy* Meals

1.

2.

3.

CHALLENGES TO REVAMPING THE HOME FOOD ENVIRONMENT

Challenge 1:

Solutions

1.

2.

Challenge 2:

Solutions

1.

2.

Challenge 3:

Solutions

1.

2.

EXERCISE THAT COULD BE DONE FOR AT LEAST 20 MINUTES
3 TIMES PER WEEK

1.

WEEK 2

TOTAL GRAMS OF CARBOHYDRATES

Sun:	Thurs:
Mon:	Fri:
Tue:	Sat:
Wed:	

NEW BRAIN-HEALTHY SNACKS TRIED AND EVALUATION OF EACH

Snack 1:

Rating (1–10):

Snack 2:

Rating (1–10):

Snack 3:

Rating (1–10):

WEEK 3

TOTAL GRAMS OF CARBOHYDRATES

Sun:	Thurs:
Mon:	Fri:
Tue:	Sat:
Wed:	

TOP 3 BRAIN-HEALTHY SNACKS

1.

2.

3.

CHALLENGES TO BRAIN-HEALTHY EATING IN THE HOME

Challenge 1:

Solutions

1.

2.

Challenge 2:

Solutions

1.

2.

Challenge 3:

Solutions

1.

2.

NEW EXERCISE THAT COULD BE DONE FOR AT LEAST **20** MINUTES **3** TIMES PER WEEK

1.

NEW BRAIN-HEALTHY SNACKS TRIED AND EVALUATION OF EACH

Snack 1:

Rating (1–10):

Snack 2:

Rating (1–10):

Snack 3:

Rating (1–10):

WEEK 4

TOTAL GRAMS OF CARBOHYDRATES

Sun:	Thurs:
Mon:	Fri:
Tue:	Sat:
Wed:	

BRAIN-HEALTHY MEALS (ASIDE FROM MEAL REPLACEMENTS) THAT COULD BE CONSUMED FOR BREAKFAST, LUNCH AND DINNER OUTSIDE THE HOME

Breakfast

1.

2.

Lunch

1.

2.

Dinner

1.

2.

BRAIN-HEALTHY MEALS THAT COULD BE ORDERED AT THE MOST FREQUENTED RESTAURANT(S) FOR BREAKFAST, LUNCH AND DINNER

Breakfast

1.

2.

Lunch

1.

2.

Dinner

1.

2.

WEEK 5

TOTAL GRAMS OF CARBOHYDRATES

Sun:	Thurs:
Mon:	Fri:
Tue:	Sat:
Wed:	

NEW EXERCISE THAT COULD BE DONE FOR AT LEAST 20 MINUTES 3 TIMES PER WEEK

1.

WEEK 6

TOTAL GRAMS OF CARBOHYDRATES

Sun:	Thurs:
Mon:	Fri:
Tue:	Sat:
Wed:	

NEW BRAIN-HEALTHY MEAL

1.

WEEK 7

TOTAL GRAMS OF CARBOHYDRATES

Sun:	Thurs:
Mon:	Fri:
Tue:	Sat:
Wed:	

WEEK 8

TOTAL GRAMS OF CARBOHYDRATES

Sun:	Thurs:
Mon:	Fri:
Tue:	Sat:
Wed:	

ENJOYMENT AND SUSTAINABILITY OF THE EXERCISES TRIED SO FAR

Exercise 1:

Enjoyment (1–10):

Sustainability (1–10):

Exercise 2:

Enjoyment (1–10):

Sustainability (1–10):

Exercise 3:

Enjoyment (1–10):

Sustainability (1–10):

WEEK 9

TOTAL GRAMS OF CARBOHYDRATES

Sun:	Thurs:
Mon:	Fri:
Tue:	Sat:
Wed:	

TOP-10 BRAIN-HEALTHY SNACKS AND MEALS EATEN OVER THE 9-WEEK PERIOD

Snacks

1.

2.

3.

4.

5.

6.

7.

8.

9.

10.

Meals

1.

2.

3.

4.

5.

6.

7.

8.

9.

10.

Proof